Health Promotion
Mobilizing Strengths to Enhance Health, Wellness, and Well-Being

Health Promotion

Mobilizing Strengths to Enhance Health, Wellness, and Well-Being

Susan Kun Leddy, RN, PhD
Professor Emerita
Widener University
Chester, Pennsylvania

F. A. DAVIS COMPANY · PHILADELPHIA

F. A. Davis Company
1915 Arch Street
Philadelphia, PA 19103
www.fadavis.com

Printed in the United States of America

Last digit indicates print number: 10 9 8 7 6 5 4 3 2 1

Publisher, Nursing: Joanne Patzek DaCunha, RN, MSN
Developmental Editor: Katherine L. Kraines
Project Editor: Tom Ciavarella

As new scientific information becomes available through basic and clinical research, recommended treatments and drug therapies undergo changes. The author(s) and publisher have done everything possible to make this book accurate, up to date, and in accord with accepted standards at the time of publication. The author(s), editors, and publisher are not responsible for errors or omissions or for consequences from application of the book, and make no warranty, expressed or implied, in regard to the contents of the book. Any practice described in this book should be applied by the reader in accordance with professional standards of care used in regard to the unique circumstances that may apply in each situation. The reader is advised always to check product information (package inserts) for changes and new information regarding dose and contraindications before administering any drug. Caution is especially urged when using new or infrequently ordered drugs.

Library of Congress Cataloging-in-Publication Data

Leddy, Susan.
  Health promotion: mobilizing strengths to enhance health, wellness, and well-being / Susan Kun Leddy.
     p. ; cm.
  ISBN-13: 978-0-8036-1405-5
  ISBN-10: 0-8036-1405-5
  1. Health promotion.   I. Title.
  [DNLM: 1. Health Promotion. 2. Health Behavior. 3. Nursing Care
  —psychology.   WA 590 L472h 2006]
  RA427.8.L43 2006
  613—dc22   2005031791

This book is dedicated to Joyce Bonaventura, RN and Raymond Vivacqua MD, "my" nurse and physician caregivers at Crozer-Medical Center in Chester, Pennsylvania.

Katherine Kraines, developmental editor for F.A. Davis, was most helpful in editing this text to make it more "user friendly." She was skilled, tactful, persistent, and gave freely of her time and effort. I am very grateful for her help.

This book originated from an "aha" I experienced when reading an article in the lay press (Fredrickson, 2003) on the value of positive emotions. The article summarized some of the insights emerging from the "positive psychology" field. This article resonated with my longstanding conceptual and theoretical interest in health as well as my frustration with the emphasis in nursing of disease diagnosis, problems, and client weaknesses. A quick search of the positive psychology literature indicated that it is vibrant and growing. Yet, paradoxically, there is almost no nursing literature on strengths (the hope literature excepted).

A number of years ago, I developed a descriptive theory of what I labeled healthiness (Leddy, 1996). This theory posited that strengths are resources for health by enhancing well-being and quality of life. The healthiness theory serves as the organizing structure for this book. Additionally, the book content serves to explicate and develop the theory. Development of an explanatory theory (Leddy & Fawcett, 1997) has been hindered by the difficulty measuring concepts such as change and energy. So, the book's content is descriptive rather than explanatory.

It is important that I emphasize the essential connectedness of all the concepts. I consider the theory to be unitary, and the separation of concepts into chapters to be artificial, and useful only for clarifying each of the concepts. For additional insight into my philosophical beliefs, the reader is encouraged to read my articles, especially (Leddy, 2003; Leddy, 2004). I have also tried very hard, (as has my developmental editor, Katherine Kraines), to move beyond conceptual and theoretical description into application to nursing practice, even in the absence of explanatory theory. Given the dearth of nursing literature to draw from, many of the "intervention strategies" originated in the psychology literature and were adapted for nursing through a retroductive process. Clearly, many of these suggestions are speculative, but appear to have face validity.

An important aspect of a strengths approach is a reconceptualization of the role of the nurse from that of an expert who knows what is best for the client, to that of the nurse as a client resource who shares power for decision-making in a relationship characterized by mutuality and genuineness. It is my fondest hope that perhaps this book will foster application of this philosophy and knowledge base in nursing practice at all levels.

Susan Kun Leddy
Summer 2005

References

Fredrickson, B. L. (2003). The value of positive emotions. *American Scientist, 91,* 330–335.

Leddy, S. K. (1996). Development and psychometric testing of the Leddy Healthiness Scale. *Research in Nursing and Health, 19,* 431–440.

Leddy, S. K., & Fawcett, J. (1997). Testing the theory of healthiness: Conceptual and methodological issues. In M. Madrid (Ed.), *Patterns of Rogerian knowing* (pp. 75–86). New York: National League for Nursing.

Leddy, S. K. (2003). A unitary energy-based nursing practice theory: Theory and application. *Visions: The Journal of Rogerian Science, 11*, 21–28.

Leddy, S. K. (2004). Human energy: A conceptual model of unitary nursing science. *Visions: The Journal of Rogerian Science, 12*, 14–27.

Nancy A. Kofoed, DNSc(c), RN
Assistant Professor, Course Coordinator
Loma Linda University
Loma Linda, California

Linda J. Patrick, RN, PhD(c)
Assistant Professor
University of Windsor
Ontairo, Canada

Sandie Soldwisch, PhD, RN, APRN-BC
Professor and NP Program Coordinator
North Park University
Chicago, Illinois

Sharon K. Stoffels, RNC, MSN
Associate Professor, Department of Nursing
Coordinator, The Idaho Hispanic Wellness Initiative: La Buena Salud
Boise State University
Boise, Idaho

Maureen Thompson, PhD, APRN
Associate Professor and Director, Nursing
College of Human Services and Health Professions
Syracuse University
Syracuse, New York

Nan Russell Yancey, PN, PhD
Associate Professor and Director of Graduate Program
Lewis University
Romeobille, Illinois

Table of Contents

Section I: The Human Strengths Approach

Chapter 1: Overview of the Human Strengths Approach, 1

Chapter 2: The Theory of Healthiness, 19

Section II: Human Strengths as Resources for Health

Chapter 3: Purpose Part One: Meaning, 31

Chapter 4: Purpose Part Two: Goals, 47

Chapter 5: Connections, 63

Chapter 6: Power Part One: Capability, 79

Chapter 7: Power Part Two: Control, 89

Chapter 8: Power Part Three: Choice, 105

Chapter 9: Power Part Four: Challenge, 111

Chapter 10: Power Part Five: Confidence, 119

Chapter 11: Power Part Six: Capacity, 131

Section III: Outcomes of Healthiness

Chapter 12: Health Strengths Outcomes, 139

Chapter 13: Health Behavior Change Theories, 155

Chapter 14: Health Behavior Change Interventions, 173

Chapter 15: A Summary of Nursing Interventions, 191

Case Studies, 203

Appendix: Leddy Healthiness Scale, 207

Index: 209

CHAPTER 1

Overview of the Human Strengths Approach

Concepts
Change

Figures & Tables
Figure 1-1 Major Health-Related
    Disciplines
Figure 1-2 Population Perspective of
    Health Promotion

Models and Theories
Intentionality: The Matrix of Healing
Broaden-and-Build Theory
Dynamical System Theories
Physiological Theories
Opponent Theory of Motivation
Dialectical Theory
Health Realization Theory
The Healthiness Theory

Interventions
Practice Model of Positive Psychological
    Assessment
The Four-Front Approach
The ROPES Model

Helpful Lists
Criteria for Strengths, pg. 9
Examples of Cultural Differences,
    pg. 11
Strategies to Enhance Cultural
    Appropriateness, pgs. 11–12
Practice Model of Positive Psychological
    Assessment, pg. 12
The Four Front Approach, pg. 13
Ways to Promote Client Strengths,
    pgs. 14–15
Health Strength Issues, pg. 15

Thought Questions
1. How does the dominant model of health differ from the model used in this book? How would you describe the relationship between strengths and health?
2. How do Western and Eastern cultures differ in their world view of the relationship between the individual and the environment?
3. What should be considered in a strengths assessment?
4. Describe the Practice Model of Positive Psychological Assessment.
5. List five ways you can promote client strengths.
6. Describe changes that are needed in nursing practice as presented in this chapter.

Chapter Synopsis
This chapter introduces the concept of human strengths as resources for health. The content addresses the nature of human strengths, and why they are important. Systems for classification of strengths and a number of human strength theories are described, stressing the importance of multicultural competency. Finally, broad assessment and intervention strategies are discussed.

Underlying the content is the belief that nursing practice must change from an exclusive focus on client problems and medical diagnoses to one including client strengths and assets as resources for health. The prevalent view of the nurse as *the* expert must be replaced with nurse-client collaborative relationships that involve the client's support system, and recognize the importance of environmental influences.

INTRODUCTION

There are two basic views of change. One view sees reality as inherently stable (seeking balance or equilibrium) and change is a threat to health and wellness. In the other view change is inevitable, stability is a momentary illusion, and reality is constantly changing. Health and wellness are considered to be dynamic, with a goal of growth and "becoming" (Overton & Reese, 1981).

The dominant model of health, consistent with the stability view, focuses on threats to health such as illness, sickness, and disease. Health is viewed as a state ranging on a continuum from an ideal state of high-level wellness to terminal illness and death. Another view suggests that health operates within a relatively narrow range of homeostatic balance, where human and environmental interactions pose potential health threats by upsetting the balance.

Alternatively, consistent with the change view, health can be understood as a single process of ups and downs, in which both disease (related to illness) and non-disease (related to wellness) are seen as complementary facets of health. Illness and wellness represent patterns of life at a particular moment. Strengths are resources that enhance health and wellness. The primary focus in this book is the promotion of positive human strengths to foster manifestations such as well-being, harmony, and growth. In the strengths model, change is inevitable and provides individuals with opportunities for growth and development. Guided by this model, the nurse focuses on changing pattern manifestations, facilitating client self-healing, and deliberately manipulating the environment to promote growth.

However, the promotion of positive resources for health does not imply that responding to threats and stressors is unimportant (Held, 2004). Both "positive" and "negative" responses can function together to move clients toward goals. For example, a woman newly diagnosed with breast cancer (negative) effectively uses her strengths (positive) to deal with the disease. Other examples of paradoxical (opposing yet complementary) views include physiological/psychological, happiness/sorrow, gain/loss, and yin/yang, in which the positive or negative evaluation depends on the individual's perspective. Because so much of the literature focuses on negative aspects of well-being and wellness, to provide balance, positive perspectives and resources are emphasized in this book.

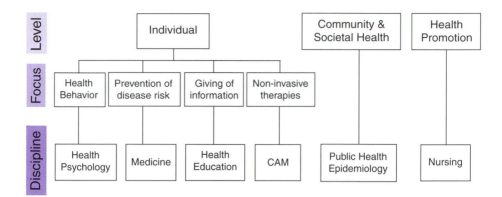

Figure 1-1. Major Health-Related Disciplines.

A number of health-related disciplines make important contributions to health promotion. These disciplines and their particular foci are indicated in Figure 1-1.

Health promotion focuses on positive health with the aim of building strengths, competencies, and resources. By identifying, acknowledging, concentrating on, and developing individual strengths and environmental resources, nurses can help improve client well-being. This requires a shift in perspective to a strengths/solution-focused, perspective-based practice rather than "reaction, coping, and repair" (Nakamura & Csikszentmihalyi, 2003, p. 262). The First International Conference on Health Promotion (held in 1986 in Ottawa Canada), promoted a positive health approach by outlining five levels of action: (1) building public health policy, (2) creating supportive environments, (3) strengthening community action, (4) developing personal skills, and (5) reorienting the health system (WHO, 1986). This book focuses primarily on developing personal skills.

Evidence indicates that depression and anxiety are prevented and good social relationships are promoted by teaching clients how and when to use their strengths, rather than focusing exclusively on repairing damage (Seligman, 2002). Feeling good makes clients more optimistic, resilient, and socially connected. Positive beliefs may be tied to physiological changes such as enhanced immune function. These beliefs may also affect physical disease by encouraging healthy behaviors, resulting in the consistent application of good health habits, and the appropriate use of health services.

Positive functioning incorporates self-acceptance, personal growth, purpose in life, environmental mastery, autonomy, and positive relationships with others including social coherence, actualization, integration, acceptance, and contribution (Keyes & Lopez, 2002). Examples of other positive attributes include courage, interpersonal skill, rationality, insight, optimism, authenticity, perseverance, realism, capacity for pleasure, future-mindedness, personal responsibility, and purpose. Interpersonal or relational attributes include patience, empathy, compassion, cooperation, tolerance, appreciation of diversity, and understanding and forgiveness (Aspinwall & Staudinger, 2003). Satisfaction of biological needs is also a strength and some theorists (e.g., Maslow) consider this to be a basic strength.

The strengths perspective significantly alters how health professionals think about their clients and the families with whom they work. It changes how nurses think about themselves, the nature of the knowledge base for practice, and the process of nursing practice itself. What is needed is an egalitarian, collaborative working relationship in a strengths/solution-based practice (Blundo, 2001). By purposefully intervening nurses can help clients anticipate future options, reflect on their ability to cope, ask questions, and use information more effectively. Through understanding the contexts that promote or hinder human strengths, nurses can assist clients to change perspective on a problem, plan a course of action, and establish better self-regulation (Aspinwall & Staudinger, 2003). Nurses can also help clients give up unattainable expectations while at the same time encouraging them to persevere toward achievable goals.

A number of overlapping terms are used in descriptions of human strengths including trait, emotion, mood, and affect. These terms will be briefly discussed.

A trait is an enduring and relatively stable characteristic that predisposes individuals for certain feelings and/or actions. For example, optimism is considered to be a trait that predisposes individuals toward hope.

Emotions are states characterized by both conscious feeling about some meaningful circumstances (i.e., they have an object), and the experience of either pleasure or pain signaling the occurrence of a beneficial or harmful event. Emotions are usually associated with experiences that can help or deter the achievement of major goals, motives, and values (Frijda, 1999). Positive emotions feel good subjectively, are brought about by favorable life conditions, and result in desirable social outcomes (Lazarus, 2003).

When individuals feel good their thinking becomes more creative, integrative, flexible, and open to information (Fredrickson, 2003). Positive emotions have also been linked to improved immune system functioning (Pettit, Kline, Gencoz, Gencoz, and Joiner, 2001), parasympathetic nervous system activation, and sufficient amounts of specific neurotransmitters (e.g., serotonin). The function of positive emotions is to facilitate active, approach behaviors through engagement with the environment.

In contrast, affect is an expression (often facial) of the feelings (emotions) associated with the awareness of pleasure or pain. It is unclear whether pleasure and pain can coexist, or are opposites, although arousal of positive affect inhibits negative affect (Frijda, 1999). However, the absence of negative affect is not evidence of positive affect.

Negative affect (NA) is associated with poor physical health, increased frequency of doctor visits, more work missed due to health concerns, lethargy, sadness, and fatigue. In contrast, positive affect (PA) is a combination of high pleasantness and high arousal, expressed as interest, engagement, and activity. High PA is a significant predictor of good health and includes feelings of interest, joy, determination, and high energy (Pettit et al., 2001).

Moods are often free-floating or objectless, relatively long-lasting, and usually follow in the wake of emotion. Since moods are based on feelings, they often predict the likelihood of successful goal-directed behavior. Negative mood is reliably associated with self-focused attention and leads to the conservation of resources and decreased involvement in the pursuit of goals. In contrast, good mood is outwardly directed and leads to increased involvement and vigorous action (Morris, 1999).

Theories help to describe and explain individual experiences. Some of the theories that relate to strengths are discussed in the following section.

HUMAN STRENGTHS THEORIES

Theories reflect a worldview and provide language and concepts to guide clinical practice. "There is no one 'best' model or theory, just as there is no 'correct' model or theory for use by every nurse in every situation" (Leddy, 2003). Nurses must first select a worldview perspective that is consistent with their philosophical beliefs (e.g., stability or change) and then identify a theory in harmony with their worldview. A model or grand theory (consistent with worldview) can provide a useful framework for selecting a theory. Nursing theories can be directly applied to practice, whereas theories from other disciplines (e.g., psychology or physiology) need to be modified for applicability to nursing practice. Several psychological, physical, and physiological theories are described in the following text.

Intentionality: The Matrix of Healing

In this nursing theory, known as IMH, intentionality is described as a "directed, purposeful mental state at the time of an act" (Zahourek, 2004, p. 41), as a "purposeful mental influence," (p. 41), and a "mental state directed toward achieving a goal" (p. 42). Intentionality is closely associated with concepts in the Healthiness Theory, such as meaning, goals, connections, choice, and capability. Intentionality is related to awareness and the appreciation for pattern, and it directs attention toward concentration and focus. The theory describes intentionality as a matrix. A matrix is defined as something from which something else "originates, develops, or takes form" (p. 46). Intentionality forms the unique environment that promotes personal healing.

The theory (IMH) proposes three developmental phases of intentionality: genetic (GI), healing (HI), and transforming (TI). GI is the potential or capacity for creating a purpose, experiencing motivation, and for initiating action, and is based largely on instinct. HI is both the capacity for and the development of a specific intent for healing. TI evolves from HI as a highly developed capacity to perceive purposeful and focused experiences, to plan and initiate action, and to formulate and initiate healing intent. In this phase, individuals "feel more connected to others and to a spiritual force or essence in the universe" (Zahourek, 2004, p. 44).

Broaden-and-Build Theory

The broaden-and-build theory (Fredrickson, 2001), a psychological theory, suggests that positive emotional experiences *expand* an individual's short-term thought-action processes, which then build long-lasting physical, intellectual, social, and psychological resources, such as the concepts in the Healthiness Theory (Fredrickson, 2001). An individual's emotional assessment of an event's meaning, initiates a sequence of responses, such as subjective experience, facial expression, cognitive processing, and physiological changes. The theory assumes that *negative emotions,* such as fear, anger, and sadness *narrow* an individual's short-term thought action processes toward quick, decisive, and specific actions. In contrast, *positive emotions,* such as joy, interest, and contentment *broaden* an individual's short-term thought-action processes, which can build enduring resources. For example, joy expands thinking through the urge to play, push the limits, and be creative. Interest grows through exploration and taking in new information and experiences. Contentment increases through the desire to savor life's circumstances and integrate them into new views of self and of the world, and pride broadens by creating the urge to share news of achievements with others and the ability to envision even greater achievements in the future (Fredrickson, 2001).

The undoing hypothesis suggests that positive emotions can undo the effect of negative emotions by expanding the narrowed psychological and physiological preparation for specific action, and triggering an "upward spiral toward enhanced emotional well-being" (Fredrickson, 2001, p. 224). This theory suggests that positive emotions can function as efficient antidotes for negative emotions.

Dynamical Systems Theory

Dynamical systems theories are based in physics and include complexity and chaos theories. Complexity theory is characterized by many independent agents interacting interconnectedly and interdependently (at all levels from individual cells to countries), spontaneous self-organization into an ecosystem with collective properties that may emerge into new properties of the system, attempts to make change advantageous, dynamism that is spontaneous rather than static (for example, a snowflake is also complicated, but it is static in form), coherent (ordered and not unpredictable as in chaos theory), and co-evolving with the environment (Anderson, Crabtree, Steele, and McDaniel, 2005; Waldrop, 1992).

Chaos theory is characterized by sensitive dependence on initial conditions, unpredictability, complex organization or structure, and non-coherence (Schuldberg, 2002). Systems can demonstrate sudden, discontinuous, and sometimes unpredictable change. Thus, "what is positive must be considered dynamic, context-dependent, and culturally and historically conditioned" (Schuldberg, 2002, pp. 337–338). This means that context and intensity determine whether personal attributes or behaviors are harmful or health promoting. Properties of dynamical systems include diversity, flexibility, many combinations and interactions, many sources of data and multiple interventions, creativity, and extended time frames (Schuldberg, 2002). Complexity and chaos theories have been used extensively to explain political and economic behavior.

Physiological Theories

A number of biochemical substances and physiological responses appear to be associated with emotions. For example, there is enhanced release of a Valium-like substance in the brain (benzodiazepine) during active behavioral coping (Drugan, 2000). In addition, dopamine levels in the brain appear to be associated with patterns of thought that are highly creative, unusual, and receptive (Fredrickson, 2000), whereas "oxytocin may mediate the benefits of positive social interaction and emotions" (Ryff & Singer, 2000, p. 38). Prolactin may also be linked with physiological effects of positive human interaction. The left frontal region of the brain is associated with positive affect and behavioral activation, and also appears to modulate immunological function in humans.

It is here hypothesized that positive emotions are associated with reduced stress-related physiological changes. This implies that positive emotions may be related to increased prefrontal activity, decreased limbic-system activity, and later changes in cortisol-mediated areas of the hippocampus and amygdala. These changes may buffer cardiovascular, immune, and cognitive and brain functioning effects of stress (Worthingon & Scherer, 2004, p. 395). In addition, there may be (a) reduced stimulation of the direct pathway from the hypothalamus to adrenals with reduction in the subsequent release of epinephrine, (b) less stimulation of the hormonally medicated HPA axis, (c) maintenance of the vagal "brake," and (d) decreased activation of the sympathetic nervous system (SNS), and engagement of the visceral afferent system. Each of these changes may lead to decreases in respiration, blood pressure, heart rate, arterial lining damage, and energy release (Worthingon & Scherer, 2004, p. 388). The research to test these hypotheses remains to be undertaken.

Neuropeptides, short strings of amino acids produced by nerve and glial cells, and their receptors form an extensive but very flexible informational network that may be the biochemical substrate of emotions (Pert, 1995). Rather than a brain-down system, Pert (1995) believes that body energies are changed by emotions, which then stimulate the release of neuropeptides throughout the body. The discovery that the same neuropeptides found in the brain are also found in immune cells (e.g., serotonin) also establishes a possible biochemical link between emotions and immunity.

Opponent Theory of Motivation

The opponent theory of motivation, a psychological theory, is based on a cyclical pattern of complimentary positive and negative emotions that are distinct in form and function (Fredrickson, 2000; Stokols, 2003). The positive-negative polarity "represents two sides of the coin of life, like structure and process, stability and change, stress and coping, and so-called positive and negative emotions" (Lazarus, 2003, p. 94).

It has been suggested that a prerequisite for cultivating personal strengths may be an exposure to negative events. When trauma is re-framed as challenge (see Chapter 9), it can transform meaning, renew faith, trust, hope, and connection. It can also redefine a sense of self and community (Ryff & Singer, 2003), and provide motivation toward enhanced well-being.

The concept of a turning point is relevant for both positive and negative events. A turning point is defined as a long-lasting redirection in an individual's life (Worthington, 2003). A turning point reflects appraisals and judgments about the direction, meaning, and circumstances of an individual's life. Personal growth often results from suffering and mastering setbacks, as well as from accomplishments and achievements (Keyes & Haidt, 2003; Worthington, 2003). For example, individuals diagnosed with cancer and other life-threatening diseases often indicate that the diagnosis resulted in a reevaluation and transformation of life's meaning and goals.

Dialectical Theory

It has been taken for granted that a state of balance, stability, and rest is more desirable than a state of upheaval, conflict, and change (stability model). However, every movement or change can be explained by the process of imbalance. In dialectics, based on philosophical theory, reality is viewed as a series of interrelating elements in a state of constant flux. All change is related to constant conflict or contradiction between opposites arising from the internal contradiction inherent in all things. But change implies potentiality, the capacity of an entity to be what it should (essence versus existence) (Betz, 1975–76; Okun, 1978). Change can resolve imbalances, contradictions, and conflicts. Crises are seen as meaningful phases in an individual's life (Riegel, 1976). In this theory, the process of transformation and development is one of opposition. However, opposites are interrelated and the meaning of one opposite is related to the other. This is known as dialectical contradiction or unity of opposites, which is distinct from mere difference or diversity.

Health Realization Theory

Health realization theory, another psychological theory, suggests that behavior can be explained as the interrelationship of three fundamental principles; thought, consciousness, and mind. Thought incorporates all mental ability. Consciousness is the sensory experience of thought as reality. And mind empowers thought and consciousness to continually merge and create experience, "Each person's mental life is a moment-to-moment product of their own thinking transformed into apparent reality by their consciousness" (Kelley, 2003, p. 52–53).

Health realization theory proposes two ways of thinking, processing-thinking and free-flowing thought. Health involves the use of both thinking styles. Because processing-thinking (e.g., critical thinking) is memory bound, individuals are limited to what they already know. In contrast, free-flowing thinking (e.g., creative thinking) "provides fresh, creative, insightful thoughts that transcend memory" (Kelley, 2003, p. 55). The occurrence of unpleasant emotions is believed to signal dysfunctional thinking.

CLASSIFICATION SYSTEMS FOR STRENGTHS

What are strengths? By looking at the contents of books that focus on strengths, it is possible to get an idea of what the authors consider to be strengths. For example, Snyder and Lopez (2003) have organized the contents of their book, *Positive Psychological Assessment; A Handbook of Models and Measures,* according to four categories: (1) cognitive; (2) emotional; (3) interpersonal; and (4) religious and philosophical models, and have also included a fifth section: positive processes, outcomes, and environments.

Peterson and Seligman (2004) provide a common vocabulary of health strengths for researchers and clinicians, which counterbalances the emphasis on disease and symptoms in the Diagnostic and Statistical Manual of Mental Disorders (DSM) sponsored by the American Psychiatric Association (1994). The overarching organizing categories in the Values in Action (VIA) classification of strengths include the core virtues of wisdom, courage, humanity, justice, temperance, and transcendence.

Character strengths define virtues. At present, 24 positive traits, or strengths, are included, such as hope, attachment, and vitality. This is the level of classification that is discussed in this book. A third level of classification includes situational themes, the "specific habits that lead people to manifest given character strengths in given situations" (Peterson & Seligman, 2003, p. 13).

Some virtues and strengths are bipolar, meaning that there is a negative anchor of the characteristic (e.g., the negative anchor for kindness is meanness). Other characteristics are seen as unipolar (e.g., humor has a zero point, but no meaningful negative anchor). Strengths may wax and wane depending on their use. This distinction has important measurement implications.

Peterson and Seligman (2003) discuss possible criteria for what they label signature strengths, these are character strengths that an individual finds fulfilling and uses often. Possible criteria for signature strengths (Peterson & Seligman, 2003) include:

- Feeling a sense of ownership and authenticity ("this is the real me").
- Feeling excited while displaying the strength, particularly at first.
- Experiencing a rapid learning curve as themes are attached to the strength and practiced.
- Yearning to act in accordance with the strength.
- Feeling unstoppable in displaying the strength. A feeling of inevitability in using the strength.
- Feeling invigorated rather than exhausted when using the strength.
- Feeling intrinsically motivated to use the strength.

Unfortunately, the future of this classification is clouded. The strengths identified through the VIA are almost completely different from those in recent compilations, and it is doubtful that a classification based on virtues will achieve widespread support.

The Healthiness Theory

The framework for the strengths discussed in this book is the Healthiness Theory (Leddy, 1996), a nursing theory, which is supplemented by numerous other conceptually related terms common in the literature (see Chapter 2).

Culture is an important factor that influences the way individuals and groups interpret and utilize strengths and weaknesses. Cultural influences are discussed in the next section and in each chapter.

MULTICULTURAL COMPETENCY

Individuals and families are embedded in a variety of sociocultural contexts or cultures, including country or region of origin, ethnicity, religion, gender, family, birth cohort, profession, politics, economics, community, prejudice, and/or discrimination. Each of these cultural contexts makes claims on the individual, and is associated with ideas and practices about how to be a "good" person (Marcus & Kitayama, 1994; Yali & Revenson, 2004).

Marcus and Kitayama (1994) view emotion as significantly enabled and shaped by cultural ideas, practices, and institutions. It is assumed that routine ways of feeling, including the tendency for emotional responses, somatic (body) experiences, or more intersubjective mood states, develop through socialization and enculturation. Core cultural values and ideals may or may not be in conscious awareness. The emotions of a given cultural group are simultaneously related to individual phenomena such as subjective affective states, facial expressions, and physiological responses. There is a collective understanding of what constitutes an individual, what is considered good or moral, and what practices support and sustain the culture (Marcus & Kitayama, 1994). As a result, "the cultural ideals and moral imperatives of a given cultural group are given life by a diverse set of customs, norms, scripts, practices, and institutions that carry out the transformation and transmission of the collective reality" (Marcus & Kitayama, 1994, p. 349).

A variety of multicultural models attempt to explain the interface between culture and human functioning, reflecting the belief that an understanding of individual behavior requires consideration of the environmental context in which it occurs (Flores & Obasi, 2003). Currently viable models include reliance on a "cultural grid," where social system variables are matched with patterns of cognitive variables. For example, cultural pluralism examines distinct cultural entities from the perspective of American values, whereas models built on human diversity assume that each individual has a unique culture (Lopez, Prosser, Edwards, Magyar-Moe, Neufeld, and Rasmussen, 2002). Some multicultural models have been discredited. For example, the inferiority model attributed variability in functioning to biological differences. This model has not been supported by research. Another discredited model, the deficit model, posited that ethnic differences were due to immutable environmental mechanisms. In contrast, culturally diverse models assume that meaning is created between relationships and events by individuals who are part of the culture (Flores & Obasi, 2003). The culturally different model means that alternative values and lifestyles are viewed as legitimate (Flores & Obasi, 2003).

Western and Eastern cultures differ in their specific or collective cultural worldview of the individual. Western cultures (e.g., the United States and Western Europe) have an independent or individualistic cultural mode emphasizing the attainment of personal happiness and fulfillment, distinguishing the self from others, making individual choices, and having personal rights. In contrast, Eastern cultures demonstrate an interdependent or collectivist cultural mode that emphasizes the self as fundamentally interrelated with others. This mode is characterized by submissiveness with dominance de-emphasized, harmoniousness in negotiated relationships, fitting in, unconditional respect, and duty to parents. "In modern Western societies, identity is personally and individually constructed. This identity must be continually verified, reexamined, updated, and defended. In more homogeneous, traditional, or Eastern cultures, identity is more closely linked to one's age, gender, status, caste, or roles; one's place in a social network is the main form of reality" (Cross & Gore, 2003, p. 544). This distinction between independent and interdependent cultural modes is an important consideration in relation to most of the strengths discussed in later chapters.

Multicultural competency requires an awareness of personal beliefs, knowledge, and skills in working with diverse populations. Nurses must understand and evaluate their own cultural frame of reference and worldview, values, prejudices, stereotypes, and reference group identity. The social-political realities, worldview, and values of cultural groups should also be identified and assessed by the nurse (Flores & Obasi, 2003).

Cross-cultural assessment includes gathering information in which the client, clinician, or researcher differ from one another by race, culture, or ethnicity. Cultural variables, such as acculturation level, racial identity, socioeconomic status, and worldview, can influence the assessment process. The nurse must understand the intricacies of culture, and be aware that every cultural group is not homogeneous. Nurses must be aware of their own biases when making constructive interpretations, and should understand that individuals may respond in what they think is a socially desirable manner, instead of giving honest answers to questions. A nurse's interpretation of the conversation should always be presented to the individual to solicit accurate feedback.

Appropriate multicultural measurement instruments must be constructed from the worldview perspective of the cultural group for which they are intended. Instruments need conceptual equivalence, meaning that the concept being measured has the same meaning for all individuals. Instruments must also be assessed for linguistic equivalence, or be administered in the preferred language of the individuals being assessed (Flores & Obasi, 2003).

Research demonstrates that although resilience, happiness, subjective well-being, and self-esteem are associated with family, group, school, and community processes across cultures, cultural differences exist. Examples of cultural differences include:

1. An orientation toward individual achievement in the United States, in contrast to Asian cultures, where social obligations and group-level accomplishments are more important (Caprara & Cervone, 2003; Lopez, Prosser et al., 2002).
2. A pretense in some cultures that life is going well, when it is not, in order to prevent placing burdens on others.
3. Doing something undesirable in some cultures reflects directly on the entire family or cultural group (Flores & Obasi, 2003).
4. In Ghanaian culture it is taboo for a child to ask how an elder is doing because the child doesn't have the wisdom to respond (Flores & Obasi, 2003).

Religious faith and spirituality are sources of emotional and social support and hope upon which disadvantaged and estranged people may be able to build strength and meaning. For example, African Americans seem to use religion for finding meaning and purpose. Additionally, the Yoruba understand that individuals have an active role in choosing their destiny and that life's obstacles may become an opportunity to work through spiritual imperfections. Within Yoruba culture, this means that the Supreme Being and departed ancestors will not abandon the person facing an unbearable task (Flores & Obasi, 2003). An important aspect of a nursing assessment includes understanding the client's personal awareness of and perspectives about spirituality. This component may affect the choices and outcomes of nursing interventions. Religion and spirituality are discussed in Chapter 3.

Common ways to enhance cultural appropriateness include peripheral, evidential, linguistic, constituent-involving strategies, sociocultural strategies, and cultural targeting and tailoring strategies (Kreuter, Lukwago, Bucholtz, Clark, and Thompson, 2002):

1. *Peripheral* strategies package health programs or materials in culturally appropriate ways, making them appealing to the target group. For example, Latinas tend to like bold and bright colors, so educational materials might be bright red.
2. *Evidential* strategies provide evidence about a particular group. For example, an evidential approach for colorectal cancer education among African Americans might include the fact that rates of colorectal cancer are higher among African Americans than other groups.
3. *Linguistic* strategies present health promotion programs and materials in the dominant or native language of the target group. This requires retaining consistent meaning and context in translation, which can be difficult.

4. *Constituent-involving* strategies draw directly on the experience of members of the target group. This may include training paraprofessionals from within the culture who can provide valuable insights into subtle cultural characteristics.
5. *Sociocultural strategies* discuss health-related issues in the context of broader social and/or cultural values and characteristics of the intended audience.
6. *Targeting* uses a single intervention approach based on characteristics shared by a particular group. There is only one version of the program or materials for all members of the group.
7. *Tailoring* attempts to reach one specific individual, based on unique characteristics identified through an individual assessment.

Although tailored approaches are intuitively attractive, it is not known whether they are more effective or cost-effective than targeted ones. When needs within a population are very similar, the variation between tailored messages will be very slight or non-existent. In this case, tailoring is unjustified. Research is ongoing to try to clarify the usefulness of these various strategies in health promotion programs.

ASSESSMENT

A strengths assessment should include: biological needs (food, shelter, and clothing); a comprehensive health assessment including physical attributes and abilities; a physical environment evaluation; a psychological evaluation (individual history, personality style and makeup, intelligence and mental abilities, self-concept and identity); a sociocultural assessment (family, friends, community, ethnicity, social, political and economic environment); and a spiritual assessment (sense of self in relation to the world, sense of meaning and purpose, value base, religious life) (Graybeat, 2001).

Practice Model of Positive Psychological Assessment

There are several approaches to assessment in the literature. The practice model of positive psychological assessment includes the following aspects (Lopez, Snyder, and Rasmussen, 2003).

1. Acknowledging the client's background, values, and biases.
2. Assuming all individuals and environments have strengths and weaknesses.
3. Conducting a comprehensive assessment.
4. Constructing an implicit theory of client functioning.
5. Gathering complementary data.
6. Testing complementary hypotheses in the context of client care.
7. Developing a flexible, comprehensive conceptualization.
8. Sharing a balanced report of the client's strengths/resources and weaknesses/deficits.

The Four Front Approach

The four front approach to data gathering and organizing identifies client attributes as follows (Lopez, Snyder et al., 2003):

1. What characteristics undermine the client? What client deficiencies contribute to the problem?
2. What are the client's strengths and assets? What strengths does the client use to deal effectively with life?
3. What needs and destructive factors are there in the environment? What environmental factors impede healthy functioning?
4. What resources and opportunities are there in the environment? What environmental resources aid positive functioning?

The ROPES Model

Another model for identifying strengths is the ROPES model (Graybeat, 2001), which stands for Resources, Opportunities, Possibilities, Exceptions, and Solutions. The model can be used as a guide for nurses to elicit client strengths. Personal and environmental factors and outcomes are linked in this model.

Environment is the individual's perception and reaction to an objective or subjective outer world. This world includes physical, social, or psychological factors that are significant to the individual (Rasmussen et al., 2003). The environment and the individual constantly influence each other and it is impossible to separate them. Thus, evaluating the individual's perception of the environment is as crucial as evaluating the actual physical and social environment (Rasmussen et al., 2003) (Figure 1-2). This assessment becomes the basis for nursing interventions.

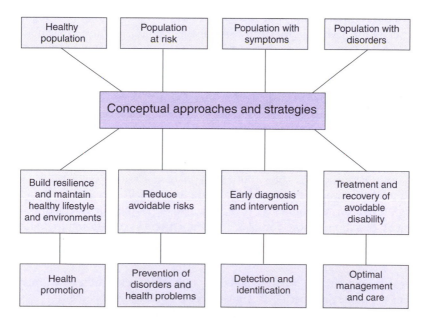

Figure 1–2. Population Perspective of Health Promotion. (Adapted from M. M. Barry (2001). Promoting positive mental health: Theoretical frameworks for practice. *International Journal of Mental Health Promotion, 3,* p. 33. Used with permission of the publisher.)

INTERVENTIONS

Traditional professional health care assumes that something about the client is broken (illness) and needs to be fixed (treatment). Within most health-related professions, including nursing, it is accepted that the expertise of the professional will make the difference in the client's life. But nursing techniques or interventions are responsible for only about 15% of the outcome (Blundo, 2001). Thus, the strengths, resilience, and social supports of the client are responsible for most of the change and how it occurs. Nurses need to understand how clients make changes and how, as nurses, they can best support each client. By doing this, the emphasis shifts from problems and deficits defined by the nurse, to possibilities and strengths identified in egalitarian, collaborative relationships with clients. This allows the client's support system and environment to move into central roles.

Blundo (2001) suggests that if nurses were able to view professional conceptualizations as hypotheses rather than facts, the basis for nursing practice could be examined from a different point of view. Questions about the client's "problem" should deliberately be eliminated from initial discussions to avoid focusing on the negative. In other words, in order to implement a strengths approach, the basic structures of practice need to be altered. "If we could focus on client strengths and assets *along with* deficits and problems, we could then design interventions *both* to decrease the weight of problems and *also to* increase the weight of assets, thereby doubling effectively altering the overall balance in a positive direction" (emphasis in the original) (Kivnick & Murray, 2001, p. 26).

A therapeutic relationship accounts for about 30% of the improvement in clients' lives (Keyes & Lopez, 2002). However, various behavioral interventions are also used, including learned optimism training, hope therapy, guided positive reappraisal, thought changing, and relaxation techniques. Learned optimism training promotes flexible thinking and resiliency by transforming negative thought into positive thought (Keyes & Lopez, 2002). Hope therapy produces creative approaches toward well thought-out goals and supplies the energy to maintain the pursuit of goals. Obstacles that appear to be insurmountable can be reframed as challenges to be overcome (Keyes & Lopez, 2002). Positive reappraisal involves focusing on the good in present and past events. Techniques for promoting emotional expression and insight include mind monitoring and thought changing, relaxation, meditation, and various imaging methods. These techniques emphasize changing states of mind rather than on manipulating external circumstances.

Relaxation therapies (e.g., meditation, yoga, progressive muscle relaxation, biofeedback, and guided imagery) cultivate feelings of contentment. Relaxation therapies also double as prevention techniques by providing practical skills for interacting with the environment, developing more complex and resilient views of self, improving immune functioning, and even extending life (Fredrickson, 2000).

Ways that the nurse can promote client strengths include:

1. Negotiating desired approaches and outcomes with clients rather than forcing them to pursue one specific outcome selected by the nurse.
2. Focusing time and money educating clients about strengths, and finding ways to build strengths rather than trying to plug skill gaps.
3. Helping clients function effectively with problems rather than trying to move them to a state of functioning without problems.

4. Paying attention to problems or pathology, while believing that solutions will come from the client's clues and creativity (Graybeat, 2001).
5. Understanding that client needs should take precedence over the charting of data. Frequently, service eligibility and reimbursement requirements reinforce a focus on client deficits.
6. Promoting certain client behaviors, while understanding that the client's motivation for the behavior can range from lack of motivation or unwillingness, to passive compliance, to active personal commitment. Nurses may be able to decrease the rate and amount of relapse by "launch[ing] people toward the state of flourishing as opposed to leaving them at the condition of languishing" (Keyes & Lopez, 2002, p. 50).

ISSUES

Aspinwall and Staudinger (2003) raise several questions and issues that stimulate discussion about human strengths:

1. How should human strengths be defined? Are strengths determined by their functionality or adaptiveness? Should subjective or objective indicators be used? Are ethical or value systems important? What criteria should be used to determine what is good or optimal?
2. Are human strengths characteristics or processes? Individuals may flexibly apply many different resources and skills to solve a problem or work toward a goal.
3. Are all strengths conscious and intentional? What strength patterns operate on an unintentional and automatic level?
4. What is the relationship between positive and negative processes? Are they interdependent or independent? Do positive strengths help individuals buffer negative events? Are positive and negative experiences reciprocal, opposite, or concurrent?
5. Is there a way to avoid assuming a value system where positive is equated with "good" and leads to prescribing what individuals should do and how they should live?
6. What are the developmental, social, and environmental contexts that influence strengths?
7. Could strengths in one situation be liabilities in another context?
8. What is the evidence that positive strengths are health resources that foster well-being and quality of life?

Many of these questions and issues will be addressed in the following chapters.

References

American Psychiatric Association. (1994). *Diagnostic and statistical manual of mental disorders* (4th ed.). Washington, DC: author.
Anderson, R. A., Crabtree, B. F., Steele, D. J., & McDaniel, R. R. (2005). Case study research: The view from complexity science. *Qualitative Health Research, 15,* 669–685.
Aspinwall, L. G., & Staudinger, U. M. (2003). A psychology of human strengths: Some central issues

of an emerging field. *A psychology of personal strengths. Fundamental questions and future directions for a positive psychology* (pp. 9–22). Washington DC: American Psychological Association.

Betz, B. R. (1975–76). A rhetoric of dialectic. *Review of Existential Psychology and Psychiatry, 14,* 129–145.

Blundo, R. (2001). Learning strengths-based practice: Challenging our personal and professional frames. *Families in Society: The Journal of Contemporary Social Services, 82,* 296–304.

Caprara, G. V., & Cervone, D. (2003). A conception of personality for a psychology of human strengths: Personality as an agentic, self-regulating system. In L. G. Aspinwall & U. M. Steudinger (Eds.), *A psychology of human strengths. Fundamental questions and future directions for a positive psychology* (pp. 61–74). Washington DC: American Psychological Association.

Cross, S. E., & Gore, J. S. (2003). Cultural models of the self. In M. R. Leary & J. P. Tangney (Eds.), *Handbook of self and identity* (pp. 536–564). New York: Guilford Press.

Drugan, R. C. (2000). The neurochemistry of stress resilience and coping: a quest for nature's own antidote to illness. In J. E. Gilham (Ed.), *The science of optimism and hope* (pp. 57–71). Philadelphia: Templeton Foundation Press.

Flores, L. Y., & Obasi, E. M. (2003). Positive psychological assessment in an increasingly diverse world. In S. J. Lopez & C. R. Snyder (Eds.), *Positive psychological assessment: A handbook of models and measures* (pp. 41–54). Washington, DC: American Psychological Association.

Fredrickson, B. L. (2000). Cultivating positive emotions to optimize health and well-being. *Prevention and Treatment, 3,* 1–25.

Fredrickson, B. L. (2001). The role of positive emotions in positive psychology: The broaden-and-build theory of positive emotions. *American Psychologist, 56,* 218–226.

Fredrickson, B. L. (2003). The value of positive emotions. *American Scientist, 91,* 330–335.

Frijda, N. H. (1999). Emotions and hedonic experience. In D. Kahneman, E. Diener, & N. Schwartz (Eds.), *Well-being: The foundations of dedonic psychology* (pp. 190–210). Washington DC: American Psychological Association.

Graybeat, C. (2001). Strengths-based social work assessment: Transforming the dominant paradigm. *Families in Society: The Journal of Contemporary Social Services, 82,* 233–242.

Held, B. S. (2004). The negative side of positive psychology. *Journal of Humanistic Psychology, 44,* 9–46.

Kelley, T. M. (2003). Health realization: A principle-based psychology of positive youth development. *Child and Youth Care Forum, 32,* 47–72.

Keyes, C. L. M., & Haidt, J. (2003). Introduction: Human flourishing. The study of that which makes life worthwhile. In C. L. M. Keyes, & J. Haidt (Eds.), *Flourishing: Positive psychology and the life well-lived* (pp. 3–12). Washington: American Psychological Association.

Keyes, C. L. M., & Lopez, S. J. (2002). Toward a science of mental health. In C. R. Snyder & S. J. Lopez (Eds.), *Handbook of positive psychology* (pp. 45–59). Oxford: Oxford University Press.

Kivnick, H. Q., & Murray, S. V. (2001). Life strengths interview guide: Assessing elder clients' strengths. *Journal of Gerontological Social Work, 34,* 7–31.

Kreuter, M. W., Lukwago, S. N., Bucholtz, D. C., Clark, E. M., & Thompson, V. S. (2002). Achieving cultural appropriateness in health promotion programs: Targeted and tailored approaches. *Health Education and Behavior, 30,* 133–146.

Lazarus, R. S. (2003). Does the positive psychology movement have legs? *Psychological Inquiry, 14,* 93–109.

Leddy, S. K. (1996). Development and psychometric testing of the Leddy Healthiness Scale. *Research in Nursing and Health, 19,* 431–440.

Leddy, S. K. (2003). *Integrative health promotion: Conceptual bases for nursing practice.* Thorofare, NJ: Slack Inc.

Lopez, S. J., Prosser, E. C., Edwards, L. M., Magyar-Moe, J. L., Neufeld, J. E., & Rasmussen, H. N.

(2002). Putting positive psychology in a multicultural context. In C. R. Snyder & S. I. Lopez (Eds.), *Handbook of positive psychology* (pp. 700–714). Oxford: Oxford University Press.

Lopez, S. J., Snyder, C. R., & Rasmussen, H. N. (2003). Striking a vital balance: Developing a complementary focus on human weakness and strength through positive psychological assessment. In S. J. Lopez & C. R. Snyder (Eds.), *Positive psychological assessment: A handbook of models and measures* (pp. 3–20). Washington, DC: American Psychological Association.

Marcus, H. R., & Kitayama, S. (1994). The cultural shaping of emotion: A conceptual framework. In. S. Kitayama & H. R. Marcus (Eds.), *Emotion and culture: Empirical studies of mutual influence* (pp. 339–351). Washington DC: American Psychological Association.

Morris, W. N. (1999). The mood system. In D. Kahneman, E. Diener, & N. Schwartz (Eds.), *Wellbeing: The foundations of hedonic psychology* (pp. 169–189). Washington, DC: American Psychological Association.

Nakamura, J., & Csikszentmihalyi, M. (2003). The motivational sources of creativity as viewed from the paradigm of positive psychology. In L. G. Aspinwall & U. M. Staudinger (Eds.), *A psychology of human strengths. Fundamental questions and future directions for a positive psychology* (pp. 257–269). Washington DC: American Psychological Association.

Okun, M. A. (1978). Implications of Riegel's dialectic approach for adult instruction. *Human Development, 21,* 316–326.

Overton, W. F., & Reese, H. W. (1981). Conceptual prerequisites for an understanding of stability-change and continuity-discontinuity. *International Journal of Behavioral Development, 4,* 99–123.

Pert, C. (1995). Neuropeptides, AIDS, and the science of mind-body healing. *Alternative Therapies in Health and Medicine, 1,* 70–76.

Peterson, C., & Seligman, M. E. P. (2003). Values in action (VIA) classification of strengths. Accessed on 10/1/03 at http://www.psych.upenn.edu/seligman/taxanomy.htm.

Peterson, C., & Seligman, M. E. P. (2004). *Character strengths and virtues: A handbook and classification.* Washington DC: American Psychological Association.

Pettit, J. W., Kline, J. P., Gencoz, T., Gencoz, F., & Joiner, T. E. (2001). Are happy people healthier? The specific role of positive affect in predicting self-reported health symptoms. *Journal of Research in Personality, 35,* 521–536.

Rassmussen, H. N., Neufield, J. E., Bouwkamp, J. C., Edwards, L. H., Ito, A., Magyar-Mae, J. L., et al. (2003). Environmental assessment: Examining influences on optimal human functioning. In S. J. Lopez & C. R Snyder (Eds.), *Positive psychological assessment: A handbook of models and measures* (pp. 443–458). Washington, D. C., American Psychological Association.

Riegel, K. F. (1976). The dialectics of human development. *American Psychologist, 31,* 689–698.

Ryff, C. D., & Singer, B. (2003). Flourishing under fire: Resilience as a prototype of the challenged thriving. In C. L. M. Keyes, & J. Haidt (Eds.), *Flourishing: Positive psychology and the life well-lived* (pp. 15–36). Washington DC: American Psychological Association.

Ryff, C. D., & Singer, B. (2000). Interpersonal flourishing: A positive health agenda for the new millennium. *Personality and Social Psychology Review, 4,* 30–44.

Schuldberg, D. (2002). Theoretical contributions of complex systems to positive psychology and health: A somewhat complicated affair. *Nonlinear Dynamics, Psychology, and Life Sciences, 6,* 335–350.

Seligman, M. E. P. (2002). Positive psychology, positive prevention, and positive therapy. In C. R. Snyder, & S. J. Lopez (Eds.), *Handbook of positive psychology* (pp. 3–9). Oxford: Oxford University Press.

Snyder, S. J., & Lopez, C. R. (2003). *Positive psychological assessment: A handbook of models and methods.* Washington DC: American Psychological Association.

Stokols, D. (2003). The ecology of human strengths. In L. G. Aspinwall & U. M. Staudinger (Eds.),

A psychology of human strengths: Fundamental questions and future directions for a positive psychology (pp. 331–343). Washington DC: American Psychological Association.

Waldrop, M. M. (1992). *Complexity: The emerging science at the edge of order and chaos.* New York: Touchstone.

World Health Organization, Health and Welfare Canada and the Canadian Public Health Association (1986). *Ottawa charter for health promotion.* Copenhagen Denmark: FADL Publishers.

Worthington, E. (2003). Turning points as opportunities for psychological growth. In C. L. M. Keyes, & J. Haidt (Eds.), *Flourishing: Positive psychology and the life well-lived* (pp. 37–53). Washington, DC: American Psychological Association.

Worthington, E. L., & Scherer, M. (2004). Forgiveness is an emotion-focused coping strategy that can reduce health risks and promote health resilience: Theory, review, and hypothesis. *Psychology and Health, 19,* 385–405.

Yali, A. M., & Revenson, T. A. (2004). How changes in population demographics will impact health psychology: Incorporating a broader notion of cultural competence into the field. *Health Psychology, 23,* 147–155.

Zahourek, R. P. (2004). Intentionality forms the matrix of healing: A theory. *Alternative Therapies in Health and Medicine, 10,* 40–49.

CHAPTER 2

The Theory of Healthiness

Concepts

Human Being (individual)
Environment
Nursing
Health
Mutual Process
Energy
Field
Self-Organization
Pattern (and Pattern Manifestations)
Awareness
Order
Change
Flexibility
Purpose
Power
Meaning
Goals
Connections

Challenge
Confidence
Capacity
Choice
Capability
Control

Figures & Tables

Figure 2-1 Energy Aspect of Universal
  Essence
Figure 2-2 The Human Energy Model
Figure 2-3 Empirically Derived
  Components of Healthiness
Figure 2-4 A Model of Healthiness
Table 2-1 Healthiness Theory Links

Models and Theories

Human Energy Model (HEM)
The Theory of Healthiness

Thought Questions

1. Can you describe the concepts and subconcepts of the Human Energy Model (HEM)? How does it compare with Rogers' Science of Unitary Human Beings (SUHB)?
2. What implications for practice do you see in the Human Energy Model?
3. The Theory of Healthiness is the structural organizer for this book. What are its major concepts and subconcepts? Do you think anything is missing? (If so, please let the author know).
4. A theory can be tested. How might you test the Theory of Healthiness?

Chapter Synopsis

This chapter presents the assumptions and constructs of the Human Energy Model (HEM) and describes the Theory of Healthiness, derived from the HEM. An available measurement instrument and research based on the theory are also reviewed. The model and theory are potentially useful for scholars and practitioners who believe in a unitary worldview, and provide an additional perspective for nurses who may be exploring available conceptual models in order to structure their practice and scholarship. Amplification of the theory of healthiness serves as the structure for this book.

Portions of the content of this chapter are reprinted with the permission of the editor, and have previously been published in *Visions: The Journal of Rogerian Scholarship* (2003), volume 11, pp. 21–28, and (2004), volume 12, pp. 14–27.

In the Human Energy Model the basis for **nursing** is a knowledge-based awareness in a goal-directed relationship with the client. The nurse-client relationship is a commitment characterized by intentionality, authenticity, mutual trust, respect, and a genuine sense of connection. "The nurse is a knowledgeable, concerned facilitator. The client is responsible for choices that influence health and healing" (Leddy, 2003, p. 68). The purpose of nursing is to facilitate harmonious pattern manifestations of both the client and nurse. Harmonious health patterning is accomplished through health pattern appraisal and recognition, and subsequent energetic interventions.

It is important to understand the Human Energy Model (HEM) in detail, because this serves as the foundation for the Theory of Healthiness. Two descriptive theories from HEM have been derived: the Theory of Healthiness and the Theory of Participation, as well as the explanatory Theory of Energetic Patterning. The first part of this chapter describes the HEM, the second part presents the Theory of Healthiness, which is discussed in detail in the following chapters.

THE HUMAN ENERGY MODEL

The HEM Worldview

The major philosophical, conceptual, and theoretical influences on the development of the Human Energy Mode (HEM) are Eastern philosophy; the vision of Martha Rogers (1970); quantum physics theory; living systems theory (Ford, 1987); process theory (Sabelli, 1989); and complexity theory (Waldrop, 1992).

The content of the HEM is grounded in the concepts of energy field; mutual human-environment process, and pattern in Rogers's (1970) Science of Unitary Human Beings; the conceptualization of health as a synthesis with illness in Newman's (1986; 1994) Theory of Health as Expanding Consciousness; and the idea of paradoxical rhythms in Parse's (1998) Theory of Human Becoming.

The View of Energy in the HEM

The HEM views everything in this world and beyond as composed of a universal essence that incorporates both particles and waves (Leddy, 2003b). "Potentiality and actuality, wave function and particle, are different phases of the same event" (Slater, 1995, p. 227). Universal essence is an undivided whole with three aspects: matter (particle), information (wave), and energy (wave). *Matter* is the potential for structure and identity, *information* is the potential for coordination and pattern, and *energy* is the potential for process, movement, and change.

Energy is defined as "the capacity to create change" (Sarter, 2002, p. 1). Changes are communicated throughout the living system (Oschman, 2000). Patterns of information for the unitary individual are provided by the coherence and timing of energy. Energy can be committed to relatively stable organizational processes, transitionally engaged in process, or can exist as free energy. Free energy can be channeled, blocked, directed, stored, accumulated and/or dissipated (Leddy, 2003b). "Energy isn't exchanged, transmitted, lost or gained; instead, it is transforming or manifesting itself eternally and in unique ways" (Todaro-Franceschi, 1999, p. 30). "Information without energy is 'powerless,' energy without information is 'purposeless' " (Schwartz & Russek, 1997b, p. 27).

The mechanism underlying energy is the vibration or oscillation of waves. "A wave is a vibrational pattern in space and time" (Capra, 1991, p. 155). Waves have a number of characteristics, including frequency, amplitude, and resonance. The number of complete vibrations that occur in a second is called the wave frequency (Jeans, 1968). "The frequency of the wave is proportional to the particle's energy" (Capra, 1991, p. 156). When wave frequency increases, wave amplitude, power, energy, and wave complexity also increase (Dardik, 1995).

In the HEM, "all forces are interactions" (Maloney, 1990, p. 386). Compatible harmonic frequencies facilitate inter-field interactions (Hunt, 1996). Resonance is the ability of a vibration to set off a similar vibration in another field, "synchronized dynamic interaction" (Schwartz & Russek, 1997a, p. 50). Oscillation of two rhythms at similar frequencies may result in vibrational coupling or locking, known as synchronization or entrainment of rhythms (Davidson, 1988; Oschman, 2000). Vibrations at similar frequencies within human and environmental fields create resonance, facilitating an increase in wave amplitude and intensity of energy (Davidson, 1988). Resonance and synchronization are the basis for the nursing energy-based interventions discussed later in this chapter.

The fundamental unit of living and nonliving systems is a field of universal essence. Rogers (1980) refers to an energy field, whereas Leddy (2003b) refers to a universal essence field. In Leddy's view energy is a part of essence, which is a larger concept. A field is described as "a domain of influence, presumed to exist in physical reality, that cannot be observed directly but that is inferred through its effects. For example, we do not actually see a magnetic field around a bar magnet; but because iron filings arrange themselves in a certain pattern, we know the field exists" (Dossey, 2000, p. 112). An energy field is a nonmaterial, dynamic web of energy interactions and transformations, with a multidimensional range of influence that coexists with the matter (physical substance) of the individual. The human being (an essence field) is embedded (networked) with interpenetrating environmental energy fields including other human beings. The individual openly participates in energy transformations with the environment, creating mutual change (Leddy, 2003a).

"Fields are known to be attracted to like fields that they resonate with; they are

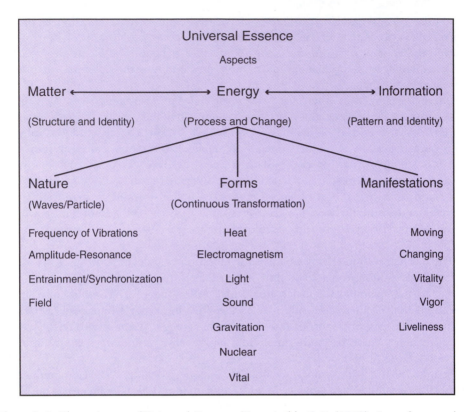

Figure 2–1. Energy Aspect of Universal Essence. (From Leddy, S. K. (2003). A nursing practice theory: Applying a unitary perspective of energy. *Visions: The Journal of Rogerian scholarship, 11,* p. 22. Used with permission.)

repulsed by those with unlike characteristics" (Hunt, 1996, p. 241). The individual's essence field can "choose" environmental patterns that resonate or interfere with self-patterning (Davidson, 1988). This happens when the individual intentionally selects and/or terminates processes with the environmental field. Imagery and therapeutic touch are interventions that are based on this principle. For example, in imagery, the client intentionally focuses on specific images from the environment. This is of clinical significance because the attentive focusing of intention may serve as a mechanism to increase frequency (and therefore intensity), complexity, and harmony of resonant energy (Schwartz & Russek, 1997b). The nature, forms, and manifestations of the energy aspect of universal essence are depicted in Figure 2-1.

HEM Concepts

The HEM, (Leddy, 2004), addresses the metaparadigm concepts of human beings, the environment, mutual human-environment process, health, and nursing. The structure of the HEM is depicted in Figure 2-2.

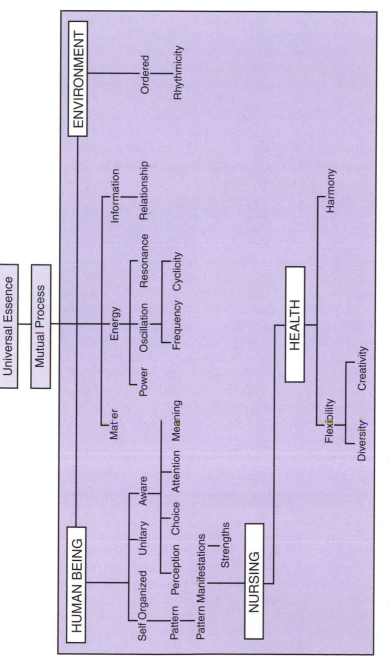

Figure 2–2. The Human Energy Model. Theories: (1) The descriptive theory of participation is derived from mutual process; (2) The explanatory theory of energetic pattern is derived from pattern manifestations; and (3) The descriptive theory of healthiness is derived from health strengths.

THE HEM CONCEPTS

Influenced by Rogers's science of unitary human beings, the **human being or individual** is viewed as a *unitary* field of universal essence that is open to and continuously interacting with an environmental universal essence field. While Rogers defined the human being as an energy field, the concept of universal essence allows the inclusion of matter and information in the field. Because everything emerges from and is embedded in essence, such divisions as body/mind/spirit, or physical/ psychological/social, are artificial analytic distinctions. The individual is *unitary,* and can only be understood as a whole.

Self-organization distinguishes the individual's universal essence field from the environmental universal essence field with which it is inseparably intermingled (Leddy, 1998). Self-organization comprises the structure of an individual. Structure is defined as "the distribution processes assumed as a consequence of the dynamic interrelations among their parts" (Fuller, 1990, p. 94). Therefore, structure is not a rigid or unchangeable framework. Self-organization is a synthesis of constancy and change that provides identity and some stability. Individuals differ in structure, but are alike in organization.

Through organization, new properties emerge unpredictably, leading to increasing diversity. However, many processes are coupled, through synchronization, so that they reoccur in particular cyclical patterned relationships (e.g., pulse and respiration, and relaxation and perception of well-being). Self-organization is demonstrated by *pattern* and its manifestations. Organized, interrelated processes form patterns. Pattern has been defined as a "configuration of relationships" (Crawford, 1982, p. 3), or as consistencies or regularities of the interconnections among energy processes. Pattern is unknowable, whereas the manifestations of pattern are accessible to human perception (in the example above, pulse rate, respiratory rate, and perception of well-being are all pattern manifestations). Because everything in the universe is in dynamic energy/matter/information transformation, constant change appears to have a sense of continuity through the recognition of patterns. What individuals perceive as stability is the relative persistence of the qualitative similarity of organized energy pattern manifestations, not a static identity (Lerner, 1984). Pattern manifestations, such as fatigue, anxiety, or pain, can be modified through energetic patterning nursing interventions, such as therapeutic touch and aromatherapy.

The individual also exhibits *awareness,* one form of energy that links the human being with the environment. Awareness makes possible perception, attention (focus), the construction of self-identity and meaning, and the ability to influence change through choice. Both separateness (analytic distinction), and holism (merging synthesis), are functions of human awareness. Through awareness, the individual perceives and categorizes pattern manifestations. These perceptions then form the basis for cognitive patterns of thinking and feeling, and intellectual patterns of determining the meaning of what is being contemplated. Therefore, meaning is a construction of human awareness and thought. Constructed meaning(s) of experience are related to purpose or goal(s) for living. Meaning has also been associated with a sense of connectedness. Through conscious choice, the individual selects, defines, modifies, and transforms experiences of participation into manifestations of diversity and harmony. This is done for example, in experiences of meaning in and of life, and the choice of long-term goals.

Environment might be regarded as the back "ground," or context, in which the individual as "the figure" is embedded (Ford, 1987, p. 51). Individuals appear distinct, but are not separate from the environment. The universal essence environment includes multiple organized units such as individuals (e.g., a nurse), family, community, or work context, and free energy embedded in its surrounding universal context.

The universal essence environment is viewed as *ordered,* demonstrating a rhythmic pattern while changing through continuous transformation of energy with matter and information. These transformations occur as a web of connectedness in relationships within the self and with the environment, including other humans and/or an "ultimate other." Change is partially unpredictable, but is also in process with an inherent order in the universe, history, pattern, and choice. Because of field order and history, there is some predictability to change, but according to quantum theory it is not possible to isolate a particular cause and effect relationship (Capra, 1991). The experience of coherence of the environment influences the individual's construction of healthiness.

Health is the pattern of the whole individual. This pattern varies rhythmically in quality and intensity over time. Health is characterized by a changing pattern of *harmony/dissonance* and diversity, which is manifested in creativity and flexibility. August-Brady (2000, p. 10) defines flexibility as an "integrative, evolving, resilient response to recognized change and uncertainty, based on openness and willingness to change, that results in a greater diversity of choice, effectiveness, and efficiency in outcomes." In contrast, this author views choice as a necessary antecedent to flexibility. Flexibility involves the openness to challenge, the will, and the ability to actively modify goals and/or behavior, as desired or needed, as the individual participates with mutual human-environmental processes.

Flexibility is not a "stand-alone" concept. This author proposes that flexibility is necessary to effectively use personal strengths. In fact, flexibility may be the pivotal quality facilitating the growth of the individual in mutual human-environment process.

Although stated at the beginning of this chapter, it is worth repeating that the basis for **nursing** is a knowledge-based awareness in a goal-directed relationship with the client. This relationship should be characterized by intentionality, authenticity, mutual trust, respect, and genuine sense of connection. "The nurse is a knowledgeable, concerned facilitator. The client is responsible for choices that influence health and healing" (Leddy, 2003a, p. 68). The purpose of nursing is to facilitate harmonious pattern manifestations of both the client and nurse that are accomplished through health pattern appraisal and recognition, and subsequent energetic interventions.

THE THEORY OF HEALTHINESS

The Theory of Healthiness forms the structural basis for this book. In this theory, health is conceptualized as a dynamic process that manifests the pattern of the unitary human being. One manifestation of health pattern is healthiness. Healthiness is defined as a process incorporating intertwined purposes, connections, and the power to achieve goals. Measurement of healthiness is therefore based on an artificial "snapshot" at a point in time. "Healthiness reflects a human being's perceived involvement in shaping change

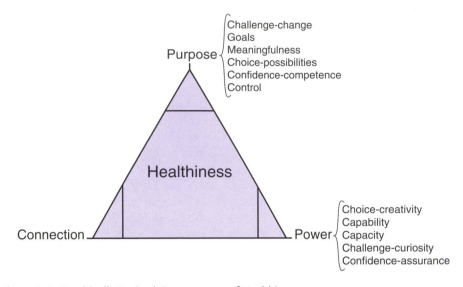

Figure 2–3. Empirically Derived Components of Healthiness

experienced in living. Therefore, healthiness is a resource that influences the ongoing pat-terning reflected in health" (Leddy, 1997, p. 49).

Purpose is defined as attributing significance and direction to the dynamic pattern of human-environment mutual process (participation). Initially, purpose was viewed as incorporating the dimensions of *meaningfulness,* defined as connections (having reward-ing relationships with others) and characterized by seeing an aspect of the present or the future as having meaning, import, or value; and *ends,* defined as goals an individual wants to reach or accomplish. However, when this descriptive theory was tested empirically, using the Leddy Healthiness Scale (LHS) (Leddy, 1996), factor analysis separated the con-nections items into a third concept, which was labeled *connections.* The revised theory is depicted in Figure 2-3.

The theory proposes that by actively channeling energy, the human being gains *power,* which is the perceived ability to direct energy toward the achievement of goals. Power incorporates the dimensions of: *challenge,* which is perceived opportunity, excitement, curiosity and/or involvement in change toward meaningful goals; *confidence,* which is an assurance of the ability to successfully overcome obstacles to achieve goals; *capacity,* which is a perceived quantity of available energy; *choice,* the perceived freedom and cre-ativity to select from among alternatives (possibilities) for action; *capability to function,* the perceived ability to work, play, and carry out activities of daily living; and *control,* which is the perceived ability to influence the rate, amount, and/or predictability of change.

The Theory of Healthiness was conceived within a unitary worldview. This means that the concepts of the theory are all networked and interconnected in reality. They have been artificially separated only for ease of discussion. Table 2-1 presents strong links among the concepts, while Figure 2-4 depicts these relationships in a graphic model.

Table 2-1. **Healthiness Theory Links**	
CONCEPT	LINKED CONCEPTS
Meaning	Goals, connections, challenge, capability
Goals	All other concepts
Connection	Meaning, goals, control, capability, confidence, choice
Choice	Goals, challenge, capability, control, capacity, confidence, connection
Challenge	Meaning, goals, choice, confidence, control
Capability	Meaning, goals, connection, choice, confidence, capacity
Confidence	Goals, connection, choice, challenge, capability
Capacity	Goals, choice, capability, control
Control	Goals, connection, choice, challenge, capacity

Empirical Research Based on the Healthiness Theory

An instrument that is consistent with the HEM is the Leddy Healthiness Scale (LHS) (Leddy, 1996). The LHS is a 26-item, 6-point Likert-type scale that measures perceived purpose, connections, and power to achieve goals. A high score indicates that the individual has significant strengths that contribute to wellness. A low score indicates fewer resources for wellness. Alpha coefficients for internal consistency reliability have ranged from 0.89 to 0.92. Test-retest reliability at 2 to 6 weeks was 0.83. The LHS is reproduced in an appendix to this chapter.

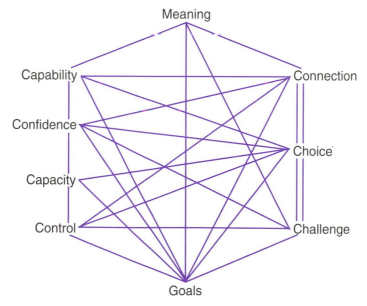

Figure 2-4. A Model of Healthiness

Using the LHS, studies (Leddy, 1996; Leddy & Fawcett, 1997) with healthy samples have demonstrated moderate to strong correlations with the Sense of Coherence Scale (Antonovsky, 1987) (r= .70), Power as Knowing Participation in Change Test (Barrett, 1986) (r= .62), Perceived Well-being Scale (Reker & Wong, 1984) (r=.74), Perceived Meaning Index (Reker, 1992) (r=.62), Person-Environment Participation Scale (Leddy, 1995) (r=.60–.73), Fatigue Experience Scale (Leddy, unpublished) (r=-.46), and the Symptom Experience Scale (Samarel et al., 1996) (r=-.54).

In a path analysis guided by a preliminary explanatory theory of healthiness (Leddy & Fawcett, 1997), participation and energy were found to have significant positive paths to healthiness, whereas change (measured as perceived stress), had a significant negative path. Energy and healthiness had significant positive paths to mental health and satisfaction with life, change had a significant negative path to current health status and a significant positive path to symptom distress, and healthiness had a significant positive path to current health status and a significant negative path to symptom distress. These data are interesting, but because of concern with the validity and appropriateness of some of the instruments, the results should be viewed with caution (Leddy & Fawcett, 1997).

References

Antonovsky, A. (1987). *Unraveling the mystery of health*. San Francisco: Jossey-Bass.

August-Brady, M. (2000). Flexibility: A concept analysis. *Nursing Forum, 35*, 5–13.

Barrett, E. A. M. (1986). A measure of power as knowing participation in change. In O. L. Strickland & C. F. Waltz (Eds.), *Measurement of nursing outcomes* (pp. 159–180). New York: Springer.

Capra, F. (1991). *The tao of physics*. Boston: Shambhala.

Crawford, G. (1982). The concept of pattern in nursing: Conceptual development and measurement. *Advances in Nursing Science, 5*, 1–6.

Dardik, I. I. (1995). The law of waves and the invalidation of the scientific method. *Cycles, 45*, 49–60.

Davidson, A. W. (1988). *Choice patterns: A theory of the human-environment relationship*. Dissertation, University of Colorado, PhD.

Dossey, L. (2000). Creativity: On intelligence, insight, and the cosmic soup. *Alternative Therapies in Health and Medicine, 6*, 12–17, 108–117.

Ford, D. H. (1987). *Humans as self-constructing living systems*. Hillsdale, NJ: Lawrence Erlbaum.

Fuller, A. R. (1990). *Insight into value*. Albany, NY: State University of New York.

Hunt, V. V. (1996). *Infinite mind: Science of the human vibrations of consciousness*. Malibu CA: Malibu Publishing.

Jeans, J. (1968). *Science and music*. New York: Dover Publications.

Leddy, S. K. (1995). Measuring mutual process: Development and psychometric testing of the person-environment participation scale. *Visions: The journal of Rogerian nursing science, 3*, 20–31.

Leddy, S. K. (1996). Development and psychometric testing of the Leddy Healthiness Scale. *Research in Nursing and Health, 19*, 431–440.

Leddy, S. K. (1997). Healthiness, fatigue, and symptom experiences in women with and without breast cancer. *Holistic Nursing Practice, 12*, 48–53.

Leddy, S. K. (1998). *Leddy and Pepper's conceptual bases of professional nursing* (4th ed.). Philadelphia: Lippincott-Raven.

Leddy. S. K. (2003a). *Integrative health promotion: Conceptual bases for nursing practice*. Thorofare, NJ: Slack.

Leddy, S. K. (2003b). A nursing practice theory: Applying a unitary perspective of energy. *Visions The Journal of Rogerian Scholarship, 11*, 21–28.

Leddy, S. K. (2004). Human energy: A conceptual model of unitary nursing science. *Visions: The Journal of Rogerian Science, 12,* 14–27.

Leddy, S. K., & Fawcett, J. (1997). Testing the theory of healthiness: Conceptual and methodological issues. In M. Madrid (Ed.), *Patterns of Rogerian knowing.* New York: National League for Nursing.

Lerner, R. M. (1984). *On the nature of human plasticity.* Cambridge: Cambridge University Press.

Maloney, D. P. (1990). Forces as interactions. *The Physics Teacher, 28,* 386–390.

Newman, M. A. (1986). *Health as expanding consciousness,* New York: National League for Nursing.

Newman, M. A. (1994). *Health as expanding consciousness* (2nd ed.). New York: National League for Nursing.

Oschman, J. L. (2000). *Energy medicine: The scientific basis.* Edinburgh: Churchill Livingstone.

Parse, R. R. (Ed.). (1998). *Illuminations: The human becoming school of thought: A perspective for nurses and other health professionals.* Thousand Oaks, CA: Sage.

Reker, G. T. (1992). *Life attitude profile manual.* Petersborough, Ontario: Student Psychologists Press.

Reker, G. T., & Wong, P. T. P. (1984). Psychological and physical well-being in the elderly. The perceived well-being scale (PWB). *Canadian Journal on Aging, 3,* 23–32.

Rogers, M. E. (1970). *An introduction to the theoretical basis of nursing.* Philadelphia: F. A. Davis.

Rogers, M. E. (1980). Nursing: A science of unitary man. In J. P. Riehl & C. Roy (Eds.), *Conceptual models for nursing practice* (2nd ed., pp. 329–331). New York: Appleton-Century-Crofts.

Sabelli, H. C. (1989). *Union of opposites: A comprehensive theory of natural and human processes.* Lawrenceville, NJ: Brunswick.

Samarel, N., Leddy, S. K., Greco, K., Cooley, M. E., Torres, S. C., Tulman, L., & Fawcett, J. (1996). Development and testing of the symptom experience scale. *Journal of Pain and Symptom Management, 12,* 221–228.

Sarter, B. (2002). *Evolutionary healing.* Boston: Jones and Bartlett.

Schwartz, G. E., & Russek, L. G. (1997a). Dynamical energy systems and modern physics: Fostering the science and spirit of complementary and alternative medicine. *Alternative Therapies, 3,* 46–56.

Schwartz, G. E., & Russek, L. G. (1997b). Information and energy in healthy systems: The soul and spirit of integrative medicine. *Advances, 13,* 25–29.

Slater, V. E. (1995). Toward an understanding of energetic healing, Part 2: Energetic processes. *Journal of Holistic Nursing, 13,* 225–238.

Todaro-Franceschi, V. (1999). *The enigma of energy: Where science and religion converge* (p. 2). New York: Crossroad Publishing.

Waldrop, M. M. (1992). *Complexity: The emerging science at the edge of order and chaos.* New York: Touchstone.

CHAPTER 3

Purpose Part One: Meaning

Concepts
Meaning
Hope

Figures & Tables
Figure 3-1 Synder's Hope Theory

Models and Theories
Parse's Human Becoming Theory
Frankl's Logotherapy
Theory of Cognitive Adaptation to
    Threatening Events
Life Experiences Model
Existential Psychology
Sense of Coherence
Maslow's Hierarchy of Needs
May's Religious Beliefs

Interventions
Cognitive-Behavioral Therapy

Meaning-Centered Counseling
Frankl's Five-Step Approach
Logotherapy Existential Psychotherapy

Helpful Lists
Sources of Meaning, pg. 33
Concepts in the Human Becoming
    Theory, pg. 34
Coping Strategies, pg. 35
Principles of The Life Experiences
    Model, pg. 36
Individual Authenticity Concepts, pg. 36
The Process of Hope, pg. 38
Components of Hope, pg. 40
Strategies for Assessing Hope,
    pgs. 40–41
Characteristics of Cognitive Behavioral
    Therapy, pg. 42
Techniques of Meaning-Centered
    Counseling, pg. 42

Thought Questions
1. Describe what specific meanings *in* life (situational meaning) and the ultimate meaning *of* life (existential meaning) mean to you.
2. Give examples of sources of meaning for you.
3. Discuss the three types of values that Frankl proposes to promote discovery of meaning. Which (if any) of these do you feel is meaningful for you?
4. What does "the silver lining of adversity" mean?
5. Compare and contrast Carver and Scheier, Seligman and Pawelski, and Snyder's approaches to hope. Which of these seems closest to your own perceptions?
6. Describe several hope assessment and intervention strategies. What would make you feel more confident about implementing these in your practice?

Chapter Synopsis

This chapter introduces the concept of meaning as an important strength and resource for health. Meaning is closely associated with the Healthiness Theory concepts of goals, connection, challenge, and capability. The content addresses various definitions about the nature of meaning, and why meaning *for* life and meaning *of* life are so important. Multiple theories related to meaning are discussed, including Frankl's logotherapy, the theory of cognitive adaptation to threatening events, the life experiences model, existential psychology, the sense of coherence, Maslow's hierarchy of needs, and May's spirituality beliefs. The related concept of hope is discussed in depth. Finally, a variety of meaning assessment and intervention strategies are proposed.

MEANING

Meaning involves comprehending words, concepts, or experiences, and understanding their significance to an individual or group. "Meaning-as-comprehensibility refers to the extent to which an event makes sense, or fits with one's view of the world (e.g., as just, controllable, and nonrandom) whereas meaning-as-significance refers to the value or worth of the event for one's life" (Davis, Nolen-Hoeksema, and Larson, 1998, p. 562). Meaning-as-comprehensibility assumes that there is order in the universe, and that negative and positive events are explainable. In contrast, meaning-as-significance has to do with life goals and purpose (Park & Folkman, 1998). Meaning described in terms of purpose refers to beliefs that organize, justify, and direct the individual. In the Healthiness Theory, goals and meaning comprise purpose. Goals constitute a central element of an individual's meaning system.

Meaning is created by individuals. Frankl (1978) wrote persuasively that there is a need for life to make sense by serving some worthy purpose. When meaning is created from experience, life is given a sense of coherence as well as purpose (King, 2004). Three common characteristics of meaning are purpose (the present has meaning because of the connection with future events), value (provides a sense that life is good and can help justify a particular course of action), and personal worth (Baumeister & Vohs, 1998). With an outcome-based perspective, meaning comes from the extrinsic things that an individual wishes to accomplish or have. In contrast, a process-oriented outlook helps an individual understand why life experiences are significant and meaningful (King, 2004).

The literature describes two different types of meaning: specific meanings *in* life (situational meaning) and the ultimate meaning *of* life (existential meaning). Situational meaning is created through the daily pursuit of life goals. Situational meaning can include finding an explanation for an event (sense-making) or finding meaning (meaning-making) by trying to understand why an event happened, what impact it had, and using reappraisal to find a positive aspect in a negative event (Schwarzer & Knoll, 2003). Behavior is directly related to the degree an individual feels important beliefs, goals, or commitments are threatened in a given situation (Park & Folkman, 1998).

In contrast, existential (global) meaning is an abstract, generalized sense that may be discovered through religious beliefs, philosophical thought, and psychological reflection

(Wong, 1998b). Wong describes existential meaning as "the need for order and coherence in the midst of chaos, the need for personal significance and self-worth in the face of entropy and death, the need for positive meanings in spite of the negative life events that often overwhelm" (Wong, 1998b, p. 396).

Life meaning can be categorized into the domains of achievement/work; relationships/intimacy; self-transcendence/generativity; and religion/spirituality. Generativity is related to activities involving the giving of self to others, or having an influence on future generations. These kinds of activities seem to result in higher levels of life satisfaction and positive affect (Emmons, 2003). Spirituality (see Chapter 5) includes the desire to establish a relationship with a transcendent dimension of reality. Intimacy, generativity, and spirituality provide more intrinsic rewards, especially when compared to actions focused on power or self-sufficiency (Emmons, 2003).

Schwarzer and Taubert (2002) suggest that cognitive, motivational, affective, relational, and personal dimensions are involved in the concept of a meaningful life. The cognitive dimension includes a belief that there is an ultimate purpose in life, moral laws, and an afterlife. Pursuing worthwhile goals, seeking to fulfill individual potential, and striving toward personal growth are examples of the motivational dimension. In the affective dimension, individuals feel content with who they are and what they are doing; feel fulfilled about accomplishments; and feel satisfied with life. The relational dimension is characterized by sincerity and honesty with others, having a number of good friends, and bringing happiness to others. The personal dimension is exemplified by enjoying challenges, accepting limitations, and having a healthy self-concept.

A number of sources of meaning have been identified including (Emmons, 2003; Wong, 1998a) the following:

1. Basic needs (food, shelter, safety)
2. Leisure activities or hobbies
3. Creative work (liking challenge, believing in and being committed to work)
4. Personal relationships (relating well and trusting others, such as family and friends)
5. Personal achievement (education or career)
6. Personal growth (wisdom or maturity)
7. Altruism (concern for the welfare of others)
8. Enduring values and ideals (truth, goodness, beauty)
9. Traditions and culture (heritage, ethno-cultural associations)
10. Legacy/generativity (contributing to society, leaving a mark for posterity)
11. Religion/spirituality (having a personal relationship with God, believing in the afterlife)

As meaning increases so does satisfaction and the sense of fulfillment (Baumeister & Vohs, 1998). "A sense that life has meaning is associated with well-being and is seen as necessary for long-term happiness" (Nakamura & Csikszentmihalyi, 2003, p. 95). Indications of meaningfulness, such as purpose in life and sense of coherence (SOC), predict positive functioning whereas indicators of meaninglessness, such as alienation and anomie, are regularly associated with psychological distress and pathology (Emmons, 2003).

MEANING MODELS AND THEORIES

Different models and theories of meaning provide "pictures" of important concepts that can be tied together in different ways. Since models and theories provide diverse perspectives, the nurse can select those representations that seem the most relevant to help guide practice and research.

Parse's Human Becoming Theory

Parse (1981) has defined nine concepts in her nursing theory. This theory is very applicable to many of the concepts in the Healthiness Theory, including meaning, choice, connection, capacity, and capability. The nine concepts are:

1. Imaging: "picturing or making real of events, ideas, and people"
2. Valuing: "living of cherished beliefs"
3. Languaging: "speaking and moving … the way one represents the structure of personal reality"
4. Connecting-separating: "the rhythmical process of distancing and relating"
5. Powering: "the pushing-resisting of inter-human encounters that originates the uniqueness in the process of transforming"
6. Transforming: "the changing of change"
7. Originating: "generating unique ways of living"
8. Revealing-concealing: "rhythmical patterns of relating with others"
9. Enabling-limiting: "infinite number of possibilities within choice."

Parse has combined these concepts into three principles. Meaning is structured multidimensionally as individuals and the environment together create (co-create) reality through "the languaging of valuing and imaging." In other words, the meaning of an individual's beliefs and values is developed and demonstrated through words and movement. The other principles are rhythmicity of patterns of relating, and cotranscendence with possibilities. Parse (1998, p. 31) says, "The unitary human being freely chooses meaning in situation, bears responsibility for the choices, and transcends with possibles."

Parse (1981) has derived three implications for practice:

1. Illuminating meaning by explicating what is appearing through language, which means describing the meaning(s) that are expressed by words.
2. Synchronizing rhythms by dwelling with the flow of connecting-separating, which means connecting with clients (and includes separation) and synchronizing with their rhythms.
3. Mobilizing transcendence by moving toward possibilities in transforming, this means moving clients toward growth and self-actualization.

Parse's theory also emphasizes presence, a way of being with the client that is open (non-routine) and without conditions. This is a qualitative method for research that is widely utilized by nursing scholars.

Frankl's Logotherapy

The three tenets of the approach to psychotherapy known as logotherapy, are the freedom of will, the will to meaning, and the meaning of life. The freedom of will liberates individuals from determinism, because they are free to choose their attitude toward the situation even though the circumstances may not change. The will to meaning is considered a primary and basic human motive. It assumes that the main goal in life is to find meaning and value through the achievement of life tasks or goals that transcend self interest rather than through goals focused on personal pleasure or power (Wong, 1998b). Finally, discovery of a meaning to life is an individual endeavor and challenge. Striving toward a valuable goal reorients an individual toward meaning, even if the search for meaning involves distress and tension.

Frankl proposed three values for discovering meaning, creative, experiential, and attitudinal. Creative values are based on the achievements and good deeds that an individual gives to the world. Experiential values refer to experiencing something or encountering someone within the environment. Attitudinal values are realized by "adopting the right attitude and taking a stand toward unavoidable suffering or an unchangeable situation" (Wong, 1998b, pp. 398–399). These values provide guidance for the nurse in helping clients clarify meaning in life.

Theory of Cognitive Adaptation to Threatening Events

According to Taylor (1983), adaptation has three main dimensions: search for meaning, sense of mastery, and self-enhancement. Understanding the cause of an event allows individuals to evaluate the event's significance and meaning. This often leads to "existential reappraisals of life and one's appreciation for it" (Schwarzer & Knoll, 2003, p. 398). Adaptation may include several coping strategies for clients, such as sense-making, benefit-finding, and benefit-reminding.

1. *Sense-making*—finding an explanation for what happened and integrating it into existing mental patterns (schema).
2. *Benefit-finding*—finding meaning by looking for the positive aspects of a negative event or the pursuit for "the silver lining of adversity" (Schwarzer & Knoll, 2003, p. 401).
3. *Benefit-reminding*—purposefully thinking about the beneficial aspects of an event in order to relieve the potentially stressful impact of a situation.

The Life Experiences Model

The life experiences model was developed within psychology and is based on motivational, developmental, and transactional elements. It is assumed that individuals have a fundamental motivation to create, engage, pursue, and maintain a sense of meaning and potential. This is true even when behavior and meaning change over the course of life under the influences of personal, interpersonal, and environmental factors. The model proposes that a sense of purpose is needed to make life worth living. A sense of purpose develops through interacting with others; taking part in leisure, work, and other activities; and through understanding oneself and the world (King, 2004).

The model has five main principles:

1. The interconnections of life experiences create a simultaneous overall experience of meaning in life.
2. The lack of predictability means that no one aspect of experience can be considered to be prior to or causal of others.
3. There are individual differences in paths to meaning, with the pursuit of belonging, meaningful activity, and understanding of meaning each linked to well-being.
4. Commitment and engagement are more fundamental to experiencing meaning in life than is the outcome.
5. Changes in meaning occur throughout life (King, 2004).

Existential Psychology

Existential psychology has several cardinal assumptions about meaning for the individual (Maddi, 1998). It is accepted that an individual's sense of meaning comes from everyday decisions and is the major determinant of thought and action. Individual authenticity is emphasized and is associated with the following concepts (Maddi, 1998):

1. Self-definition is the ability to understand and influence social and biological experiences.
2. Functioning shows "directional change, innovativeness, and continuity over time" (Maddi, 1998, p. 13).
3. Changes can create opportunities as the individual seeks a broader perspective, deeper understanding, and takes decisive actions (Maddi, 1998).
4. Biological and social experiences show subtlety, taste, intimacy, and love.
5. Ontological anxiety (or doubt) though frequent, is a natural part of creating meaning and does not undermine the decision-making process (Maddi, 1998).
6. Ontological guilt (or sense of missed opportunity) is minimized.
7. Experiences of failure are accepted as natural and provide learning opportunities (Maddi, 1998).
8. Experiential evaluation emphasizes that an experience is positive if it fits into the individual's life pattern. Nothing can be expected to last forever.

When there is an emphasis on past experience, current experiences are seen as givens or unshakable truths. In other words, the past is seen as dictating the future, leaving individuals with few options in making present choices. In order for individuals to make choices based on what is possible, they must look toward the future rather than basing choices on past experience (Maddi, 1998). Unfortunately, few individuals have sufficient existential courage (self-confidence and self-reliance) to tolerate the uncertainty of regularly choosing the future.

Sense of Coherence

The sense of coherence (Antonovsky, 1987) comprises comprehensibility, manageability, and meaningfulness. Comprehensibility refers to a belief that the universe is predictable, ordered, and makes "cognitive sense." Manageability is the belief that individuals possess the personal and social resources to confront and deal with demands. Meaningfulness, the most significant component of a sense of coherence, refers to the degree to which an individual's life makes emotional sense, with life demands seen as worthy of energy and commitment (Korotkov, 1998). These concepts are perceived as generalized resources for resisting stress, and therefore are presumed to promote health.

Maslow's Hierarchy of Needs

Maslow (1968) proposed that individual needs form a hierarchy, with some needs taking precedence over others. The higher individuals move up on the hierarchy of needs the more meaningful their lives become (Wong, 1998b). Physiological needs (e.g., oxygen, water, and food) are the most basic of survival needs (deficit needs or D-needs). Next are the needs for safety and security (e.g., safety, stability, and protection), love and belonging (e.g., friends, affection, and community), and finally, esteem (e.g., status, respect of others, and self-respect). If survival needs are met, the being need for self-actualization (B-need) becomes a priority. Self-actualization is the continuous desire to fulfill personal potential. Under stressful conditions or when survival is threatened an individual may "regress" to a lower need level.

Maslow's theory has been criticized because of lack of scientific rigor in development of his conception of self-actualization, and evidence that indicates that many individuals strive toward self-actualization even when their basic needs are unfulfilled. For example, artists such as Rembrandt, van Gogh, and Toulouse Lautrec, all suffered from poverty while creating their timeless masterpieces. Despite these criticisms however, Maslow's theory still is influential in nursing.

May

May (1940), who wrote extensively on religion, believes that the essence of religion is the belief that something matters, the presumption that life has meaning. He also emphasized making choices and being authentic as ways of experiencing meaning. Personal meaning is derived from consciously making and committing to decisions. The courage to maintain individuality and self-acceptance determine authenticity (Wong, 1998c).

A concept related to meaning is hope, which is discussed in the following section.

RELATED CONCEPTS

Hope

There are three major approaches to hope in the literature. Carver and Scheier (2002) discuss dispositional optimism, which is the expectation that good things will be plentiful in the future and that bad things will be scarce. This approach requires that clients set and try to meet goals. However, optimism (see Chapter 4) is regarded as a separate (rather than interchangeable) concept by most theorists. Seligman and Pawelski (2003) describe the explanatory style, which attributes bad events to external, unstable, and specific causes. This approach also values agency, the belief that goals can be achieved. The third approach, advanced by Snyder (2000), states that hope includes agency and pathways (plans to meet goals).

Hope is "characterized by a confident yet uncertain expectation of achieving a future good which, to the hoping person, is realistically possible and personally significant" (Dufault & Martocchio, 1985, p. 380). Hope involves anticipation combined with thinking, acting, feeling, and relating, and is directed toward a personally meaningful future fulfillment (Stephenson, 1991). Consequently, action is an inherent component of hope-mustering energy. However, the intensity of hope is not dependent on whether the goal is actually attainable but does depend on the individual's subjective sense of confidence or doubt about a goal's attainability (expectancy-value framework) (Morse & Duberneck, 1995). Hope is a relatively stable characteristic, which may be essential for life (Stephenson, 1991).

Generalized hope is broad in scope, is not linked to any particular concrete or abstract object, and is a sense of some future unknown beneficial development. In contrast, particularized hope is concerned with a hope object, a particularly valued outcome, good, or state of being. Objects of hope may be concrete or abstract, explicitly stated or implied (Dufault & Martocchio, 1985).

According to Stephenson (1991) the process of hope involves thinking about and visualizing something that does not yet exist. After an object of hope is identified, there is an estimation of the probability of certain outcomes. "The person searches for clues to provide the grounding for hope [and]... as long as the individual believes that a foundation is present upon which hope rests assurance will be felt" (Stephenson, 1991, p. 1458). Positive feelings and a sense of confidence usually exist, and even when diluted by uncertainty hope seems to strengthen, empower, and energize the individual.

International studies of hope were conducted in nine countries, guided by the Human Becoming Theory (Parse, 1981; 1998) and using the Parse research methodology. It was found that structures of hope consistently included anticipation of possibilities in the face of adversity, arduous difficulties, and ambiguity (Parse, 1999).

Snyder, Irving, and Anderson (1991, p. 287) define hope as "a positive motivational state that is based on an interactively derived sense of successful (a) agency (goal-directed energy), and (b) pathways (planning to meet goals)." Agency is the motivational component encouraging individuals to pursue their goals. Pathways tap abilities to plan realistic routes to goals, and create multiple ways to work around barriers.

According to Snyder and colleagues (2001), the process of hope can be understood through the following activities:

1. Obtaining the client's learning history with particular attention to dispositional agency (capacity) and pathways (plans).
2. Evaluating the goal outcome. In other words, is the potential outcome important enough for the individual to sustain agency and pathways? It needs to be of "sufficient magnitude to command sustained attention" (p. 104).
3. Enhancing agency and pathway components as they interact with each other.
4. Achieving the goal/or not. Since perceptions about success in pursuing goals drives emotion, it is important to obtain emotional feedback.
5. Sustaining or changing levels of hope over time.

Rather than an emotion-based process, hope is considered by these authors to be a cognitive process with emotional correlates and outcomes (Lopez, Floyd, Ulvan, and Snyder, 2000). Emotions are thus considered a by-product of goal-directed thought (Snyder, 2000). Hope refers to the future, in contrast to well-being which refers to the recent past

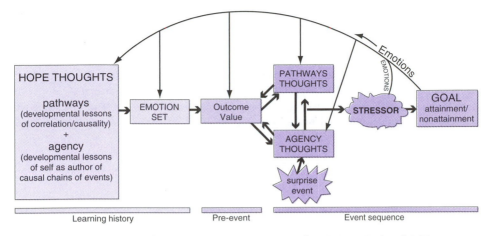

Figure 3–1. Synder's Hope Theory. (From Lopez, S. J., Snyder, C. R., & Pedrotti, J. T. (2003). Hope. Many definitions, many measures. In S. J. Lopez & C. R. Snyder (Eds.), *Positive psychological assessment: A handbook of models and measures* (p. 96). Washington DC: American Psychological Association. Copyright 2003 by the American Psychological Association. Reprinted with permission.)

(Magaletta & Oliver, 1999). According to Snyder and colleagues (2001), hope utilizes both pathways and agency thinking. Pathways thinking is characterized by a sense of being able to generate successful plans and alternative routes to meet goals (ways). The essential motivation required to use alternative routes is agency thinking, the capacity to use pathways to reach desired goals (will) (Magaletta & Oliver, 1999; Snyder, Rand, and Sigman, 2003).

Six dimensions of hope have been identified: affective, cognitive, behavioral, affiliative, temporal, and contextual. The *affective* dimension focuses on the sensations and emotions involved in the hoping process. Nurses can foster this dimension by allowing clients to express how and why hope is important to them. Clients should feel free to share the wide range of emotions associated with hope, including feelings of both confidence and uncertainty. The nurse should convey an empathetic understanding of the client's worries, fears, and doubts and try to alleviate these feelings when possible. By encouraging endurance, courage, and patience the nurse can help clients avoid feeling immobilized by their feelings.

The *cognitive* dimension focuses on how individuals wish, imagine, wonder, perceive, think, remember, learn, generalize, interpret, and judge in relation to hope. High-hope individuals appraise their goals positively and as a challenge (Lopez, Ciarletti, Coffman, Stone, and Wyatt, 2000). Nurses can support this dimension by helping clients clarify and modify their perceptions of reality. The *behavioral* dimension focuses on actions, such as organizing ideas, planning strategies, and making decisions. This dimension also includes thinking about how to resolve a situation or how to create a climate where hope might be fulfilled. The nurse can focus on enhancing the client's self-esteem and capabilities with the goal of diminishing feelings of helplessness.

The *affiliative* dimension focuses on the individual's sense of other-centered involvement and relatedness. This dimension includes social interaction, mutuality, attachment, and intimacy, other-directedness, and self-transcendence. The nurse can promote this dimension by encouraging clients to talk about goals related to life, dying, and death, and by giving clients opportunities to readjust plans and reminisce. The *temporal* dimension focuses on the experience of time and includes the degree to which the past, present, and future are part of the hoping process, and whether hope is time dependent. The *contextual* dimension focuses on those life situations that surround and influence hope.

Based on a study of hope (Morse & Duberneck, 1995) in patients waiting for heart transplants (hoping for a chance for a chance); spinal cord-injured patients (hoping for incremental gains); breast cancer survivors (hoping against hope); and breastfeeding working mothers (provisional hope, based on finding alternatives to solve problems), Morse and Duberneck (1995, p. 278) identified what they consider to be universal components of hope. However, these components were based on understanding hope as a response to a threat, which is an example of particularized hope. The universal components of hope that they identified include:

1. Assessing the predicament or threat realistically
2. Picturing alternatives and the setting of goals
3. Bracing for negative outcomes
4. Making a realistic assessment of personal and external resources
5. Soliciting mutually supportive relationships
6. Evaluating continuously for signs that reinforce the selected goals
7. Determining to endure

Post-White (2003) describes what she labels as common attributes of hope, which include relying on personal inner resources; living in the present moment; and having positive expectations, goals, and a future orientation. Correlates of hope include connectedness and support from family, friends and health-care professionals; and spiritual and religious beliefs and practices. Outcomes of hope may include finding meaning, restored optimism, a sense of confidence, valuing of meaningful relationships, and appreciating each day.

Research has identified positive correlations between hope and the belief in personal capabilities, feelings of self-worth and self-esteem, lower levels of depression in children, positive thinking and affect, increased achievement performance (academic and athletic), problem-solving, and coping with illness-related problems (Snyder, Sympson, Michael, and Cheavens, 2001). Hope has a strong relationship with well-being and life satisfaction (Snyder, 2004). Hope has also been related to better adjustment to chronic illness, severe injury, and handicaps, making contact with other individuals, more social support, more social competence, and less loneliness. No gender differences in hope have been found in more than 40 studies.

Assessment of Hope

King (2004, pp. 87–88) identifies a number of strategies for the assessment of hope. These strategies can be used by nurses and include:

1. Looking for articles that are symbolic of the client's interests (e.g., objects in the environment important to or expressive of the client).
2. Gathering information about activities valued by the client (e.g., the things they most like to do, their family or personal rituals, and things they celebrate or take pride in).
3. Inviting clients to tell their life story, communicate their concerns and spiritual

needs, and hopes and dreams. Talking with them about their habits and rituals and why they are important.

4. Allowing clients to express their concerns or needs about their sense of meaning in life by using questionnaires or activities (e.g., therapeutic play and forms of artistic impression).

5. Asking open-ended questions to:
   a. Discover how important belonging, doing, and understanding are to clients.
   b. Determine whether clients can articulate their goals and needs about belonging, doing, and understanding.
   c. Determine why the client's specific goals for therapy intervention are important (i.e., determine the meaning of the goals). Will they help the client attain a sense of belonging, competence, or understanding?

6. Assessing the strengths and resources of clients and their families with respect to knowledge, abilities, or skills. Assess the resources and support needed for clients to engage in the three spheres of life, which are belonging, doing, and understanding, by:
   a. Determining the client's degree of self-knowledge and self-efficacy (or comfort level) in the domain of interest.
   b. Determining the client's strengths and competencies (and self-awareness with respect to these).
   c. Determining the client's knowledge of recreational and vocational opportunities in the community.
   d. Assessing family factors, such as financial resources and time availability.
   e. Assessing external supports, such as existing friendships and other informal social supports.

Assessment is fostered by using discovery-oriented interview questions in a collaborative nurse-client relationship that includes the client's support system, and recognizes the importance of environmental influences. This approach also helps the nurse facilitate the client's development of meaning and hope through various interventions.

Interventions to Facilitate Development of Meaning and Hope

A number of interventions encourage the development of hope including: hope-reminding (of previous successful hope endeavors), narrative hope-finding (strands of hope that run throughout life), hope-bonding (formation of a sound therapeutic alliance characterized by personal attachment, mutual trust, and respect), and increasing the positive rather than decreasing the negative (Lopez, Floyd, et al., 2000). Interventions that aid in the development of meaning, include cognitive-behavioral therapy, meaning-centered counseling, Frankl's five-step approach, and logotherapy.

Cognitive-Behavioral Therapy (CBT)

The process-related characteristics of cognitive-behavioral therapy are that (Taylor, Feldman, Saunders, and Illardi, 2000, p. 111):

1. Therapy is brief, directive, and collaborative.
2. The frequent use of Socratic questioning is used as a teaching-learning device.
3. Goals are defined and prioritized.

4. The issues are addressed hierarchically with current functioning and behaviors first, followed by cognitive patterns and schemata. Relapse prevention is emphasized at the end of therapy.

Cognitive-behavioral therapy goals are implemented within a treatment protocol and a therapeutic relationship. The goals are (Michael, Taylor, and Cheavens, 2000, p. 156):

1. Removing goal blockages
2. Increasing agency and providing effective pathways to desired goals
3. Helping clients to let go of unattainable goals and substitute new ones
4. Achieving symptom remission, which is the primary goal (Taylor et al., 2000, p. 113)
5. Dealing with solutions to problems rather than the problems themselves

The goals of CBT are met through its content and intervention strategies. Nurses need to be comfortable in encouraging the expression of and responding to issues of meaning, including spiritual issues (King, 2004). It is also important to understand the cultural differences of clients and their families. Examples of content in CBT include giving a verbatim, convincing, and explicit rationale; assigning homework; and giving and eliciting feedback about progress toward treatment goals. Strategies to facilitate goals include creating a hierarchy of goals divided into small manageable goals; behavioral techniques, such as scheduled mastery and pleasure activities, cognitive rehearsal, self-reliance training, role-playing, in vivo exposure, worry exposure, relaxation training, time management, and problem-solving; and cognitive therapies, such as hypnosis, reality testing, self-monitoring, and identifying and modifying of cognitive distortions (Taylor et al., 2000, p. 112).

Meaning-Centered Counseling

Some techniques that are suggested for nurses using a meaning-centered approach include (King, 2004):

1. *Contextualizing the problem*—placing the problem in the context of the client's present and overall life situation.
2. *Attributional probing*—revealing the deep reasons for the client's problems, such as faulty assumptions, distorted self-defeating attitudes, unresolved existential conflicts.
3. *Life review* and play back.
4. *Fast-forwarding*—depicting likely scenarios given a particular choice.
5. *Magical thinking*—transcending present thinking (if clients had the freedom and money to do whatever they wanted on a daily basis, what would it be?).
6. *Constructing a personal meaning profile*—components are religion, positive relationships, achievement, self-transcendence, self-acceptable, meaning and purpose, self-realization.
7. *Targeting and contracting*—attainable goals by completing assignments or practicing new skills.
8. *Effective coping*—accepting life's realities and learning to see positive meanings in negative life events.

9. *Overcoming the Achilles' heel*—clients are their own worst enemies; self-destructive; something is holding them back from developing their full potential.
10. *Promoting belonging*—social support (e.g., support groups, clubs, drop-in programs).
11. *Promoting competency* and providing feedback about skill level (e.g., involvement in sports and recreation programs; volunteer and paid employment experiences).
12. *Promoting self-awareness* (e.g., self-discovery programs, values clarification exercises and workshops).
13. *Providing instruction* in the fundamental skills needed for belonging (e.g., programs that assist the client in developing proactive social skills).
14. *Listening* to the concerns and issues of the client.
15. *Considering* ways to bring about desired goals.
16. *Referring* clients to pastoral staff and qualified counselors to assist with issues concerning spirituality, belonging, and vocational guidance.
17. *Encouraging* creative expression and personal style in the performance of everyday activities.
18. *Focusing* on goals, obstacles, alternative routes to goals, and determination in pursuit of goals (Michael et al., 2000).
19. *Using language* and examples, or visual aids and activities that fit clients' abilities to comprehend and express themselves.

Frankl's Five-Step Approach

Frankl developed a five-step approach to meaning therapy that is practiced by Lukas at the Viktor Frankl Institute for Southern Germany, in Furstenfeldbruck (cited in Fabry, 1998). The steps in the approach are:

1. Defining the problem
2. Finding the areas of freedom where there are choices
3. Listing available choices
4. Identifying which choice has the most meaningful response among the available choices
5. Doing something to bring about the meaningful response

Logotherapy Existential Psychotherapy

Frankl also developed logotherapy (Frankl, 1992), a process of psychotherapy that is based on existential psychology. Logotherapy helps the client to find meaning in life, even if it requires change. "When we are unable to change a situation, we are challenged to change ourselves" (Frankl, 1978, p. 39). Two of the major concepts of logotherapy include paradoxical intention, and deflection. In paradoxical intention, fear brings about the very thing that is feared. Forced intention makes it impossible to avoid the fear and therefore exaggerates uncontrollable symptoms. To bring symptoms under volitional control, the approach promotes doing the opposite of what the client is afraid of (e.g., if the client is afraid of sleep, try to stay awake). In deflection, clients who are excessively preoccupied with their own painful emotions are encouraged to concentrate on external circumstances in order to focus outside themselves (Maddi, 1998). Logotherapy should only be used by nurses with special training. It is an especially useful intervention for use by psychiatric nurse practitioners.

References

Antonovsky, A. (1987). *Unraveling the mystery of health: How people manage stress and stay well.* San Francisco: Jossey-Bass.

Baumeister, R. F., & Vohs, K. D. (1998). The pursuit of meaningfulness in life. In P. T. P. Wong & P. S. Fry (Eds.), *The human quest for meaning: A handbook of psychological research and clinical applications* (pp. 608–618). Mahwah, NJ: Lawrence Erlbaum.

Carver, C. S., & Scheier, M. F. (2002). Optimism. In C. R. Snyder, & S. J. Lopez (Eds.), *Handbook of positive psychology* (pp. 231–243). Oxford: Oxford University Press.

Davis, C. G., Nolen-Hoeksema, S., & Larson, J. (1998). Making sense of loss and benefiting from the experience: Two construals of meaning. *Journal of Personality and Social Psychology, 75,* 561–574.

Dufault, K., & Martocchio, B. C. (1985). Hope: Its spheres and dimensions. *Nursing Clinics of North America, 20,* 379–391.

Emmons, R. A. (2003). Personal goals, life meaning, and virtue: Wellsprings of a positive life. In C. L. M. Keyes, & J. Haidt (Eds.), *Flourishing: Positive psychology and the life well-lived* (pp. 105–123). Washington DC: American Psychological Association.

Fabry, J. (1998). The calls of meaning. In P. T. P. Wong & P. S. Fry (Eds.), *The human quest for meaning* (pp. 295–305). Mahwah, NJ: Lawrence Erlbaum.

Frankl, V. E. (1978). *The unheard cry for meaning. Psychotherapy and humanism.* New York: Simon & Schuster.

Frankl, V. E. (1992). *Man's search for meaning. An introduction to logotherapy* (4th ed.). Boston: Beacon Press.

King, G. A. (2004). The meaning of life experiences: Application of a meta-model to rehabilitation sciences and services. *American Journal of Orthopsychiatry, 74,* 73–84.

Korotkov, D. (1998). The sense of coherence: Making sense out of chaos. In P. T. Wong & P. S. Fry (Eds.), *The human quest for meaning: A handbook of psychological research and clinical applications* (pp. 51–70). Mahwah, NJ: Lawrence Erlbaum.

Lopez, S. J., Floyd, R. K., Ulvan, J. C., & Snyder, C. R. (2000). Hope therapy: Helping clients build a house of hope. In C.R. Snyder, *Handbook of hope: Theory, measures and applications* (pp. 123–150). San Diego: Academic Press.

Lopez, S. J., Ciarletti, R., Coffman, L., Stone, M., & Wyatt, L. (2000). Diagnosing for strengths: On measuring hope building blocks. In C. R. Snyder, *Handbook of hope: Theory, measures and applications* (pp. 57–85). San Diego, CA: Academic Press.

Maddi, S. R. (1998). Creating meaning through making decisions. In P. T. P. Wong & Fry, P. S (Eds.), *The human quest for meaning: A handbook of psychological research and clinical applications* (pp. 3–26). Mahwah, NJ: Lawrence Erlbaum.

Magaletta, P. R., & Oliver, J. M. (1999). The hope construct, will and ways: Their relations with self-efficiency, optimism, and general well-being. *Journal of Clinical Psychology, 55,* 539–551.

Maslow, A. H. (1968). *Toward a psychology of being* (2nd ed.). New York: Harper & Row.

May, R. (1940). *The springs of creative living: A study of human nature and God.* New York: Abingdon-Cokesbury.

Michael, S. T., Taylor, J. D., & Cheavens, J. (2000). Hope theory as applied to brief treatments: Problem-solving and solution-focused therapies. In C.R. Snyder (Ed.), *Handbook of hope: Theory, measures and applications* (pp. 151–166). San Diego, CA: Academic Press.

Morse, J. M., & Duberneck, B. (1995). Delineating the concept of hope. *Image: Journal of Nursing Scholarship, 27,* 277–285.

Nakamura, J., & Csikszentmihalyi, M. (2003). The construction of meaning through vital engagement. In C. L. M. Keyes & J. Haidt (Eds.), *Flourishing: Positive psychology and the life well-lived* (pp. 83–104). Washington DC: American Psychological Association.

Park, C. L. & Folkman, S. (1998). Meaning in the context of stress and coping. *Review of General Psychology, 1,* 115–144.

Parse, R. R. (1981). *Man-living-health: A theory of nursing.* New York: Wiley.

Parse, R. R. (1998). *The human becoming school of thought.* Thousand Oaks, CA: Sage.

Parse, R. R. (1999). *Hope: An international human becoming perspective.* Sudbury, MA: Jones & Bartlett.

Post-White, J. (2003). How hope affects healing. *Creative Nursing, 1,* 10–11.

Schwarzer, R., & Knoll, N. (2003). Positive coping: Mastering demands and searching for meaning. In S. J. Lopez, & C. R. Snyder (Eds.), *Positive psychological assessment: A handbook of models and measures* (pp. 393–409). Washington DC: American Psychological Association.

Schwarzer, R., & Taubert, S. (2002). Tenacious goal pursuits and striving toward personal growth. In E. Frydenberg (Ed.), *Beyond coping: Meeting goals, visions, and challenges* (pp. 19–35). Oxford: Oxford University Press.

Seligman, M. E. P., & Pawelski, J. O. (2003). Positive psychology: FAQs. *Psychological Inquiry, 14,* 159–163.

Snyder, C. R. (2004). Hope and the other strengths: Lessons from *Animal Farm. Journal of Social and Clinical Psychology, 23,* 624–627.

Snyder, C. R. (2000). *Handbook of hope: Theory, measures and applications.* San Diego, CA: Academic Press.

Snyder, C. R., Irving, L., & Anderson, J. R. (1991). Hope and health: Measuring the will and the ways. In C. R. Snyder, & D. R. Forsyth (Eds.), *Handbook of social and clinical psychology: The health perspective* (pp. 285–305). Elmsford, NY: Pergamon.

Snyder, C. R., Rand, K. L., & Sigman, D. R. (2003). Hope theory. In C. R. Snyder, & S. J. Lopez (Eds.), *Handbook of positive psychology* (pp. 257–276). Oxford: Oxford University Press.

Snyder, C. R., Sympson, S. C., Michael, S. T., & Cheavens, J. (2001). Optimism and hope constructs: Variants on a positive expectancy theme. In E.C. Chang (Ed.), *Optimism and pessimism: Implications for theory, research, and practice* (pp. 101–125). Washington DC: American Psychological Association.

Stephenson, C. (1991). The concept of hope revisited for nursing. *Journal of Advanced Nursing, 16,* 1456–1461.

Taylor, J. D., Feldman, D. B., Saunders, R. S., & Illardi, S. S. (2000). Hope therapy and cognitive-behavioral therapies. In C. R. Snyder (Ed.), *Handbook of hope: Theory, measures and applications.* San Diego, CA: Academic Press.

Taylor, S. E. (1983). Adjustment to threatening events: A theory of cognitive adaptation. *American Psychologist, 38,* 1161–1173.

Wong, P. T. P. (1998a). Meaning and successful aging. In I. B. Weiner, (Ed.), *The human quest for meaning: A handbook of psychological research and clinical applications* (pp. 359–394). Mahwah, NJ: Lawrence Erlbaum.

Wong, P. T. P. (1998b). Meaning-centered counseling. In P. T. P. Wong & P. S. Fry (Eds.), *The human quest for meaning: A handbook of psychological research and clinical applications* (pp. 395–435). Mahwah, NJ: Lawrence Erlbaum.

Wong, P. T. P. (1998c). Implicit theories of meaningful life and the development of the personal meaning profile. In P. T. P. Wong & P. S. Fry (Eds.), *The human quest for meaning: A handbook of psychological research and clinical applications* (pp. 112–139). Mahwah, NJ: Lawrence Erlbaum.

CHAPTER 4

Purpose Part Two: Goals

Concepts
Optimism
Flow

Figures & Tables
Figure 4-1 Self-Concordance Model
Table 4-1 Common Cognitive Distortions

Models and Theories
King's Theory of Goal Attainment
Self-Concordance Model
Self-Determination Model

Interventions
Beck's Cognitive Therapy
Optimism Training

Helpful Lists
Strategies for Addressing Unattainable
    Goals, pg. 50
Characteristics of Flow, pg. 51
Hypotheses from King's Theory of Goal
    Attainment, pg. 52
Mechanisms Linking Optimism and
    Health, pg. 57
Interventions to Foster Optimism,
    pg. 58
Strategies to Promote Goal Attainment,
    pg. 59
Intervention Dos and Don'ts,
    pg. 59

Thought Questions
1. What are the roles of goals in promoting health?
2. What is the relationship between goals and values?
3. How would you differentiate between intrinsic/extrinsic and approach/ avoidance goals?
4. What are five cognitive distortions that clients might exhibit? What are possible implications for nursing interventions?
5. How do differences between types of optimism affect nursing interventions?
6. Which nursing intervention dos and don'ts seem most important to you? Why?

Chapter Synopsis
This chapter introduces the concept of goals as a resource for health, and establishes why planning and action toward fulfilling goals are important. Goals are related to all of the other concepts in the Healthiness Theory. The related concept of optimism is discussed. Several goal theories are described, including King's goal attainment theory, the self-concordance model, self-determination theory, and Beck's cognitive therapy. The importance of multicultural competency is stressed, and intervention strategies are discussed.

GOALS

Much of the literature about goals, grounded in the stability model of change, is based on expectancy-value models of motivation. These models suggest that effort toward a goal requires confidence in eventually achieving the goal (expectancy), and that the goal matters to the individual (value) (Carver & Scheier, 2003). Thus, optimism leads to confidence about successful outcomes, resulting in persistent effort to accomplish goals.

"To be lived well, life must have purpose" (Ryff & Singer, 1998, p. 216). Goals structure life and add purpose, reflect core values, and are associated with pursuits that give meaning and dignity to daily existence. Goals can compensate for feelings of inferiority, provide meaning in the present and give hope for the future, and help realize individual potential. Goals that provide purpose in life and personal growth are characteristic features of and contributors to health (Griffith & Graham, 2004; Ryff & Singer, 1998).

Goals are actions, conditions, or values that are either desirable or undesirable. Meaningful goals motivate and energize individuals to act. Commitment is "the belief that the goal is important and the belief that one can achieve or make progress toward it" (Locke, 2003, p. 305). Thus, commitment overlaps with agency, the belief that goals can be achieved. Self-enhancement goals include those oriented toward achievement, agency, and power. Group-enhancement goals include affiliation, intimacy, communion, relatedness, and interpersonal connection. Global-enhancement goals embrace protecting the environment, improving the quality of life of all people, and eradicating crime and war (Schmuck & Sheldon, 2001).

Values are achieved by pursuing goals and over a lifetime individuals undertake multiple values and goals. But prioritizing values is critical to managing life, both now and in the future (Locke, 2003). Emotions provide the energy and motivation to act and serve as rewards for successful actions or inducements to avoid painful ones. For example, the author of this book strongly values scholarly productivity. Consequently, completing this manuscript was the accomplishment of a valued goal, resulting in feelings of satisfaction, gratification, and pleasure, making the achievement feel even more meaningful. "Emotional intensity reflects subconscious perceived value, threat, or achievement as well as the value in one's value hierarchy" (Locke, 2003, p. 302). In the absence of emotion, values are experienced as dry, abstract, and intellectual.

Individuals perform best when goals are both specific and difficult (Locke, 2003). Goals can also be differentiated by their level of abstraction from concrete to abstract. In the example above, scholarly productivity is an abstract goal, whereas the completion of a specific book manuscript is a concrete goal. The discrepancy between input and reference value determines approach or avoidance goals. Approach goals reduce discrepancy and avoidance goals increase differences. For example, a consistent and disciplined writing schedule is an approach strategy that provides positive feedback about progress toward a valued goal. Sporadic or infrequent writing is an avoidance strategy that increases the discrepancy between the goal and progress toward its achievement. Goals vary in importance, with higher level goals (i.e., finding meaning in life vs. a decision about what to eat for dinner) usually more important. Goals can be described as intrinsic (internally driven) or extrinsic (externally driven) in origin.

Individuals are inclined toward activity and integration, but they also are vulnerable to passivity. Thus, motivation is a critical variable in producing and maintaining change (Ryan & Deci, 2000). Intrinsic motivation is an innate tendency to seek out novelty and challenge, to extend and exercise individual capacities, explore, learn, and achieve personal growth and happiness, have meaningful relationships, and make a contribution to society (Bauer & McAdams, 2004; Ryan & Deci, 2000). Intrinsic motivation can be increased by encouraging clients to be self-directed, make choices, and to acknowledge feelings. Things that diminish intrinsic motivation include tangible rewards, threats, deadlines, directives, pressured evaluations, and imposed goals. External regulation, an example of extrinsic motivation from individuals or groups, is associated with less interest in, valuing of, and effort toward achievement; a concern for money, status, possessions, and physical appearance; and a tendency to avoid responsibility for negative outcomes (Bauer & McAdams, 2004). Extrinsic motivation results in decreased levels of growth and well-being (Griffith & Graham, 2004).

The advantages of intrinsic motivation appear to be considerable, including more effective behavior, increased persistence, good feelings, and being part of a social group. Critically important for intrinsic motivation to occur are relatedness, which is the need to belong and to connect with others, perceived competence, and autonomy. The nurse can increase the client's internal motivation by facilitating choice, volition, and freedom from excessive external pressure toward behaving or thinking a certain way. For example, variations in these components have independently predicted the level of daily well-being among nursing home residents. How satisfied employees were with their experiences of autonomy, competence, and relatedness in the workplace predicted their performance and well-being at work (Ryan & Deci, 2000).

Individuals who are authentically motivated show more interest, excitement, and confidence. These qualities are experienced as enhanced performance, persistence, and creativity, and as heightened vitality, self-esteem, and general well-being. The advantages of greater internalization include "more behavioral effectiveness, greater volitional persistence, enhanced subjective well-being, and better assimilation of the individual within his or her social group" (Ryan & Deci, 2000, p. 73). The achievement of intrinsic goals aids well-being, whereas the imposition of extrinsic goals provides little benefit.

Approach goals focus on moving toward or maintaining a desirable or positive outcome. In contrast, avoidance goals focus on moving away from or inhibiting an undesirable or negative outcome (Dickson & MacLeod, 2004). Avoidance goals are associated with less positive psychological outcomes than approach efforts. Avoidance efforts place individuals at risk for emotional and physical "ill-being" (Emmons, 2003). Thus, it is more effective for the nurse to encourage clients to work toward positive goals than to avoid negative goals. When a goal is unattainable there are two options, remain committed to the goal and experience distress or dissolve the commitment and disengage from the goal. According to Carver and Scheier (2003, p. 92), disengagement has four potential patterns. These patterns can be used by nurses to help clients deal with unattainable goals:

1. *Choosing an alternative path*—if the alternative has the same value as the original goal, positive outcomes and feelings are possible.
2. *Choosing a new goal*—positive outcomes and feelings are also possible.
3. *Scaling back aspirations*—positive outcomes and feelings are possible.
4. *Giving up* a goal without establishing a new one results in feelings of helplessness. "Real helplessness occurs when a goal cannot be reached and also cannot be abandoned, because it matters too much" (p. 90).

Goal engagement is facilitated by adopting a new goal, taking a new path toward an existing goal, or scaling back aspirations and adopting a more realistic goal. Being unable to disengage from unattainable goals can negatively affect well-being, particularly in older adults (Scheier & Carver, 2003). Because flexibility promotes health the nurse can be a source of support and encouragement in helping clients adjust their goals and flex with the circumstances.

Disengagement consists of at least two components, reduced effort and a decrease in the value attached to the goal. Reducing effort and commitment frees up personal resources, which can have beneficial effects in other areas of life. For example, an individual with arthritis might substitute machine quilting for hand quilting, or seek another creative activity (e.g., photography, drawing), instead of wasting energy railing against an insurmountable physical hardship. Therefore, when helping clients disengage from unattainable goals, the nurse should offer alternative meaningful goals. Both goal disengagement and goal re-engagement have been independently related to indicators of well-being, such as high purpose in life, low intrusive thoughts, low perceived stress, and high self-mastery (Wrosch & Scheier, 2003).

A meaningful purpose in life and a sense of personal growth promote immune competence and increase activation in the left prefrontal region of the cerebrum, which is associated with a disposition toward a positive affect. (Ryff & Singer, 1998). Empirical evidence also indicates that meaning in life and positive emotions help to restore an individual's worldview and may build additional personal resources (Schwarzer & Knoll, 2003). However, short-term goals that are necessary for daily functioning contribute little to the sense that life is meaningful.

Csikszentmihalyi (1990) developed the concept of flow to describe a goal-oriented experience. Flow is characterized by vitality, intensity, and a felt connection to the goal. Individuals actively engaged with the environment form goals, selectively focus attention, and then construct the meaning of their experience. "Vital engagement is participation in an enduring relationship that is enjoyed and meaningful" (Nakamura & Csikszentmihalyi, 2003, p. 83).

The flow state is developed by clear, immediate goals, continuous and unambiguous feedback about progress, and opportunities that stretch existing capabilities. Entering flow depends on establishing a balance between perceived capacities and perceived challenges. Characteristics of flow include:

1. Intense and focused concentration on the present.
2. A loss of self-consciousness as action and awareness merge.
3. A sense of being able to handle the situation because of knowing how to respond to whatever will happen next.

4. A sense that time has passed more quickly or slowly than normal.
5. An experience of the activity as rewarding in and of itself, regardless of the outcome (Nakamura & Csikszentmihalyi, 2003).

Coping is a second concept involved with goal pursuit. Coping can be thought of as a continuum extending from flourishing in the pursuit of successful goals to the management of stress and adaptation (Frydenberg, 2002). Assimilative coping is the attempt to adjust ongoing life circumstances to match personal goals, needs and desires (adjust circumstances to goals). For example, an individual who wants to write a story, may turn down an invitation to attend a movie in order to work toward his or her goal. In contrast, accommodative coping adjusts personal preferences and goals to the constraints of the situation (adjust goals to circumstances) (Carver & Scheier, 2003). Therefore, the individual may postpone writing a first draft of an article because they have not obtained the necessary information from the library. Much of the literature on coping focuses on the management of stress at the negative end of the continuum, but recently there has been some discussion of proactive coping at the positive end of the continuum. Proactive coping is discussed in Chapter 9.

Self-efficacy (task-specific self-confidence) is a third strategy associated with goal-setting. "People with higher self-efficacy set more difficult goals for themselves, are more likely to be committed to difficult goals that are assigned, are more likely to sustain their efforts after negative feedback, and are more likely to discover successful task strategies than people with lower self-efficacy" (Locke, 2003). The main ways to build efficacy are through training and practice, observing others through role-modeling, and persuasive encouragement.

In the absence of specific goals an individual's performance will not usually improve, even with feedback. In other words, vague goals produce vague actions. Goal achievement can also be blocked by irrationally putting wishes ahead of reality; being unwilling to think and work hard; and being controlled by fear that focuses on avoiding loss. However, Locke (2003, p. 310) observes that "those who live only to avoid hurt are the living dead." The pursuit of meaningful goals is essential for meaning and purpose in life.

GOAL THEORIES

King's Theory of Goal Attainment

Guided by her systems interaction model, King (1987; 1995) developed a nursing theory of goal attainment. A critical concept in the theory is mutual goal-setting, "a shared collaborative process in which client and nurse give information to each other, identify goals, and explore means to attain goals, each moves forward to attain goals" (King, 1989, p. 155). From the theory, a transaction process model has been designed to lead to goal attainment when practiced (King, 1989).

Examples of testable hypotheses generated from King's theory include the following (King, 1987, p. 111):

1. Mutual goal-setting will increase the client's functional abilities in performing activities of daily living.
2. Goal attainment will be greater in clients who participate in mutual goal-setting than in clients who do not participate.
3. Role conflict between nurse and client may increase stress in the nursing situation.

Self-Concordance Model

The self-concordance model (Fig. 4-1) addresses the alignment of needs with motivation, not an easy objective. Self-concordant goals are inspired by developing interests and deeply felt personal values (Sheldon, 2001). Needs are considered to be both motives and required inputs and serve to energize, reward, and reinforce particular behaviors (Sheldon, 2001).

Individuals strive for meaning by using proactive processes. "Selecting goals which correctly represent 'who one really is' presumably requires complex self-perceptual abilities, in which one must take account of one's current situation, one's unfolding interests, one's deeper beliefs, and one's longer-term needs" (Sheldon, 2001, p. 22). Goals must represent the client's underlying interests and values, otherwise, deeper needs may go unmet. It is important for individuals to know their enduring values and interests in order to resist squandering motivational energy on dead-ends or blind alleys. Clients must differentiate between personal goals and those interests and values established by others. By asking questions nurses can often help clients clarify their goals.

An individual might select nonconcordant goals (1) by assimilating conformist or even harmful impulses from the environment; (2) because of deficiencies in level of ego- or identity-development; (3) due to fears about giving up known behavior (even if the behavior is not satisfying); and (4) by wanting to maintain positive social feedback, even if it is not ultimately conducive to self-development. In contrast, positive effects of self-concordance include (1) prediction of concurrent well-being and greater well-being after goals are attained; and (2) prediction of effort and goal attainment.

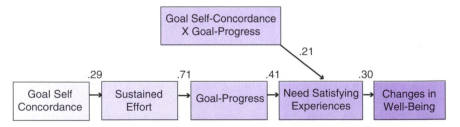

Figure 4–1. Self-Concordance Model. (From Sheldon, K.M. (2001). The self-concordance model of healthy goal striving: When goals correctly represent the person. In P. Schmuck & K. M. Shelton (Eds.), *Life goals and well-being: Towards a positive psychology of human striving* (p. 24). Seattle, WA: Hogrefe & Huber.)

Self-Determination Theory

Self-determination theory focuses on the social-contextual conditions that support self-motivation and health development, and highlight the importance of evolved inner resources for growth. Motivation involves energy, direction, and persistence (Ryan & Deci, 2000). The theory proposes that three innate psychological needs—competence (see Chapter 6), autonomy (see Chapter 7), and relatedness (see Chapter 5)—enhance self-motivation and health.

Beck's Cognitive Therapy

Beck's (1995) cognitive therapy is based on the interactions among cognition, affect, and behavior. Automatic thoughts are immediate and related to a spontaneous appraisal of the situation. Appraisal, in turn, elicits and shapes an emotional and behavioral response. Schemas are also an integral part of this approach. Schemas comprise interrelated concepts, beliefs, and assumptions that are automatically activated ("the way things are"); interpersonal strategies; and may include persistent misperceptions of situations that result in errors of reasoning. Common cognitive distortions are listed in Table 4-1.

Table 4-1. **Common Cognitive Distortions**

DISTORTION	DEFINITION
Dichotomous thinking	Viewing experiences in terms of two mutually exclusive categories with no "shades of gray" in between. For example, believing that one is *either* a success *or* a failure and that anything short of a perfect performance is a total failure.
Overgeneralization	Perceiving a particular event as being characteristic of life in general rather than as being one event among many. For example, concluding that an inconsiderate response from one's spouse shows that she doesn't care despite her having showed consideration on other occasions.
Selective abstraction	Focusing on one aspect of a complex situation to the exclusion of other relevant aspects of that situation. For example, focusing on the one negative comment in a performance evaluation received at work and overlooking the positive comments.

(continued on following page)

Table 4-1. **Common Cognitive Distortions** *(Continued)*

DISTORTION	DEFINITION
Disqualifying the positive	Discounting positive experiences that would conflict with the individual's negative views. For example, rejecting positive feedback from friends and colleagues on the grounds that "they're only saying that to be nice," rather than considering whether the feedback could be valid.
Mind reading	Assuming that one knows what others are thinking or how others are reacting despite having little or no evidence. For example, thinking, "I just know he thought I was an idiot!" despite the other person's having given no apparent indication of his reactions.
Fortune telling	Reacting as though expectations about future events are established facts rather than recognizing them as fears, hopes, or predictions. For example, thinking "He's leaving me, I just know it!" and acting as though this is definitely true.
Catastrophizing	Treating actual or anticipated negative events as intolerable catastrophes rather than seeing them in perspective. For example, thinking, "Oh my God, what if I faint!" without considering that although fainting may be unpleasant or embarrassing, it is not terribly dangerous.
Maximization and minimization	Treating some aspects of the situation, personal characteristics, or experiences as trivial and others as very important, independent of their actual significance. For example, thinking "Sure, I'm good at my job, but so what, my parents don't respect me."
Emotional reasoning	Assuming that one's emotional reactions necessarily reflect the true situation. For example, concluding that because one feels hopeless, the situation must really be hopeless.
"Should" statements	The use of "should" and "have to" statements that are not actually true to provide motivation or control over one's behavior. For example, thinking "I shouldn't feel aggravated. She's my mother, I have to listen to her."

(continued on following page)

DISTORTION	DEFINITION
Labeling	Attaching a global label to oneself rather than referring to specific events or actions. For example, thinking "I'm a failure!" rather than "Boy, I blew that one!"
Personalization	Assuming that one is the cause of a particular external event when, in fact, other factors are responsible. For example, thinking, "She wasn't very friendly today, she must be mad at me," without considering that factors other than one's own behavior may be affecting the other individual's mood.

Source: From Pretzer, J.L. & Walsh, C. A. (2001). Optimism, pessimism, and psycho therapy. In E.C. Chang (Ed.), *Optimism and pessimism: Implications for theory, research, and practice* (p. 326). Washington, DC: American Psychological Association. Copyright 2001 by the American Psychological Association. Reprinted with permission.

Pretzer and Walsh (2001) describe a number of interventions designed to increase positive thinking, or at least achieve a balance between positive and negative thinking. But a decrease in negative thinking does not necessarily increase positive thinking.

A concept related to goals is optimism, which is discussed in the following section.

RELATED CONCEPTS

Optimism

Optimism is a particular generalized expectancy that good things will happen in life (Carver & Scheier, 2001). Expectancy-value theories emphasize the psychological anticipation of the future and assume that behavior is aimed at the pursuit of goals. Expectancies are beliefs that due to either personal effort or other factors beyond the individual's control, desired outcomes will occur (Magaletta & Oliver, 1999).

Optimism is defined as "a relatively stable, generalized expectation that good outcomes will occur across important life domains" (Wrosch & Scheier, 2003, p. 64). Optimism is simply the belief that good future outcomes will occur (an expectation), whereas personal control refers to the belief that individuals bring about desired outcomes through their own efforts (an attribution) (Aspinwall & Brunhart, 2000). Optimism is sometimes confused with beliefs about personal control, but there are clear empirical and conceptual differences between attributions and expectations (Garber, 2000). Individuals who have confidence about the future tend to continue their efforts, even when dealing with serious problems (Scheier, Carver, and Bridges, 2002), whereas pessimism leads to passivity.

Dispositional Optimism

Dispositional optimism refers to generalized positive expectations about future events. Optimists and pessimists use different strategies to manage critical life situations. Dispositional optimists tend to persist in pursuing their goals because they make more favorable appraisals of successfully meeting goals. More active and less avoidant ways of coping with stress may mediate the psychological benefits associated with dispositional optimism (Aspinwall & Brunhart, 2000). Individuals who are confident about their future exert continuing effort, even when dealing with serious problems. They tend to use more problem-focused coping strategies, and when problem-focused coping is not possible, optimists turn to adaptive emotion-focused coping strategies, such as acceptance, use of humor, and positive reframing (Wrosch & Scheier, 2003). Consequently, dispositional optimism has beneficial effects on well-being and health.

Individuals with high scores on measures of dispositional optimism, meaning that their general expectations are positive, report fewer depressive symptoms, greater use of effective coping strategies, and fewer physical symptoms than do pessimistic individuals (Gillham, Shatte, Reivich, and Seligman, 2001). "Optimism is positively correlated with the vigor with which the immune system responds to an antigen challenge" (Peterson, & Bossio, 2001, p. 136). Optimists may use more adaptive health habits and use them more often (Mulkana & Hailey, 2001). Optimists perceived themselves to be in better health and tended to describe their health more positively (Bosompra, Ashikaga, Worden, and Flynn, 2001). But individuals with an optimistic bias and dispositional optimism may also neglect their health (thinking they are healthier than they are) and consequently have more health issues (Peterson & Chang, 2001).

Explanatory Style

The explanatory style is the characteristic way an individual explains earlier events based on internal vs. external causes, stable vs. unstable occurrences, and global vs. specific causes. "People are optimistic when they attribute problems in their lives to temporary, specific, and external events as opposed to permanent, pervasive, and internal causes (Reivich & Gillham, 2003, p. 59). Beliefs about events may be accurate, inaccurate, or difficult to determine.

An adult's explanatory style is usually stable but can change. Positive thinking is powerful because it sets into motion a complex cascade of biological, psychological, and social processes that promote health (Peterson & Bossio, 2001). An optimistic explanatory style is associated with higher levels of well-being, motivation, and achievement, and lower levels of depression (Gillham et al., 2001). In contrast, a pessimistic explanatory style is associated with self-defeating behaviors reflecting a tendency to seek distraction from unpleasantness or to give up (Carver & Scheier, 2002). However, pessimism is not always dysfunctional—it depends on the context. For example, a pessimistic perspective may help an individual give up pursuing an unachievable goal.

It is unclear whether optimism and pessimism are endpoints of a single continuum or two separate concepts with distinct effects (Aspinwall & Brunhart, 2000). Scheier, Carver, and Bridges (2002) consider optimism and pessimism to be polar opposites on a one-dimensional continuum. However, according to Peterson and Chang (2001), optimism and pessimism are not simple opposites. Positive and negative thought content are nearly uncorrelated (Garber, 2000; Riskind, Sarampote, and Mercier, 1996), and decreasing negative thinking does not necessarily increase positive thinking (Pretzer & Walsh, 2001). Individuals can be low, medium, or high in negative thinking, regardless of their levels of positive thinking (Riskind et al., 1996). Therefore, the nurse can help clients achieve a balance between positive and negative thinking by encouraging positive thinking, decreasing negative thinking, and increasing realistic thinking, mindfulness, and acceptance.

When dealing with difficulties in their lives, optimists experience less distress than pessimists (Carver & Scheier, 2002). Optimists tend to use problem-focused coping and positive reframing, especially when the stressful situation is viewed as controllable. They are also inclined to accept the reality of a situation even when it is seen as uncontrollable. Optimism is associated with active, problem-solving coping, instead of denying and distancing from the problem. Optimists turn to strategies such as acceptance when there are specific health threats and problem-focused coping is not a possibility. Acceptance of threats such as serious disease keeps the individual engaged with goals and life (Carver & Scheier, 2002).

Optimism predicts good health with moderate correlations on "self-report, to physician ratings of general well-being, to doctor visits, to survival time following a heart attack, to immunological efficiency, to successful completion of rehabilitation programs, and finally to longevity" (Peterson, 2000, p. 149). Optimism can also decrease the likelihood of an initial onset of illness; it can decrease the severity of illness; speed recovery; and make relapse less likely (Peterson, 2000). Mechanisms linking optimism and health include (Peterson, 2000, pp. 151–152):

1. *Immunological pathways*—"optimism correlates positively with a vigorous immune system response to an antigen challenge" (Peterson, 2000, p. 151).
2. *Emotional pathways*—optimism is incompatible with depression.
3. *Cognitive pathways*—there is a belief that good health can be maintained and promoted with fewer complications.
4. *Social pathways*—individual action is promoted.
5. *Behavioral pathways*—"healthy" practices must be vigorous and sustained.

MULTICULTURAL COMPETENCY

The conception, appropriateness, selection, and achievement of personal goals are affected by ethnic group membership, cultural orientation, family of origin, socioeconomic status, political and religious affiliations, gender, age, heredity, and level of education, to name a few of many variables (Griffith & Graham, 2004).

Europeans and North Americans tend toward individualism, which includes the valuing of personal happiness and fulfillment, an independent self, individual choices, and personal rights. Eastern cultures see the self as fundamentally interrelated with others; and stress submissiveness with dominance deemphasized; harmoniousness; fitting in; and unconditional respect and duty to parents. Asian Americans are significantly more pessimistic, but are not less optimistic than white Americans. Asian Americans use more problem avoidance and social withdrawal strategies to deal with stressful situations (Chang, 2001). The nurse's understanding of the cultural background of a client helps to determine or modify appropriate interventions

INTERVENTIONS

Nursing interventions can increase optimism, decrease pessimism, or both. The client plays an active role in developing an understanding of the problems and in the change process. The client and nurse work together (Pretzer & Walsh, 2001). The nurse should intervene flexibly, rather than in a "cookbook" fashion, by tailoring interactions and goals to the needs of each client. The nurse can increase the motivation for change by helping clients identify the costs of pessimism and the benefits of optimism. The nurse should also check for fears about possible consequences of change, such as having to give up habitual routines. Identifying and challenging pessimistic thoughts involves helping clients to critically evaluate their thoughts and draw realistic conclusions. However, optimism may not be increased by decreasing pessimism. Identified alternatives to pessimism should be relatively easy to believe (e.g., learning to suspend judgment or assessing the reasonableness of feelings); result in beneficial changes in mood and behavior; be practical to implement in real-life situations; and be likely to be supported by experience in real life. One approach that has been used to try to increase optimism is optimism training.

Optimism Training

Optimism training can be defined "as the use of cognitive techniques that are explicitly intended to enhance positive thinking and optimistic thought content" (Riskind et al., 1996, p. 106). The key factor in treatment success and psychological well-being is the enhancement of positive thinking.

A study with 83 undergraduate college students aged 18 to 36 years old yielded a positive picture, with 4 of 5 dependent measures (optimistic interpretation, positive cognition, problem-solving self-efficacy, and word generation) significantly improved by optimism training. There was no effect on negative thinking. The following interventions can be used by nurses to promote realistic thinking and acceptance, mindfulness, and optimism.

1. Have the client maintain a daily diary to document how they are doing and how their thinking is changing.
2. Have the client identify and modify dysfunctional optimism that leads to unrealistic thinking, and identify beneficial alternative views.
3. Encourage positive visualization to identify problems and ways of coping. This can include "story boarding," which involves picturing scenes leading to a desired outcome, and "invulnerability training," promoting good feelings about how a particular situation was handled.
4. Consider using the "silver lining" technique to try to find a positive benefit in a negative experience.
5. Consider using "pump priming," in which clients note experiences relevant to the patterns they want to encourage or change.

6. An "anti-procrastination sheet" can be completed by the client expressing how difficult or how rewarding it will be to perform a task, including the best, worst, and most likely outcomes.

Relapse prevention should plan for high-risk situations including practicing coping skills.

Further nursing strategies to promote goal attainment include (Griffith & Graham, 2004):

1. Using relaxation, meditation, and stress management skills to help in the management of negative affect (NA).
2. Helping clients use direct (assertive) but also respectful communication of their needs and desires so others can understand and decide whether or not they can accommodate requests.
3. Using active listening to understand and interpret accurately the client's message.
4. Being present while probing for a deeper understanding and paraphrasing back what was heard.
5. Using problem-solving and task-management strategies.

Intervention Dos and Don'ts

Some specific dos and don'ts for helping clients in optimism interventions include the following suggestions (Lopez, Floyd, Ulvan, and Snyder, 2000).
DO

- Break a long-range goal into steps or subgoals.
- Begin to pursue a distant goal by concentrating on short-term goals.
- Practice planning different routes to goals and select the best one.
- Mentally practice the actions needed to accomplish the goal.
- Mentally rehearse scripts about how to react in the event of a blockage.
- When a goal is not reached, conclude that the strategy was unworkable, don't self-blame.
- If a new skill is necessary to reach the goal, learn it.
- Cultivate two-way friendships, be willing to give and receive advice.
- Be willing to ask for help in reaching a desired goal.

DON'T

- Think big goals can be accomplished all at once.
- Be too hurried in producing routes to goals.
- Be rushed to select the best or first route to the goal.
- Over analyze with the idea of finding one perfect route to the goal.
- Stop thinking about alternate strategies when one doesn't work.
- Self-blame when an initial strategy fails.
- Be caught off guard when one approach doesn't work.
- Get into friendships where there is praise for not coming up with solutions to problems.

References

Aspinwall, L. G., & Brunhart, S. M. (2000). What I do know won't hurt me: Optimism, attention to negative information, coping, and health. In J. E. Gilham (Ed.), *The science of optimism and hope* (pp. 163–200). Philadelphia: Templeton Foundation Press.

Bauer, J. J., & Mc Adams, D. P. (2004). Growth goals, maturity, and well-being. *Developmental Psychology, 40,* 114–127.

Beck, J. S. (1995). *Cognitive therapy: Basics and beyond.* New York: Guilford Press.

Bosompra, K., Ashikaga, T., Worden, J. K., & Flynn, B. S. (2001). Is more optimism associated with better health? Findings from a population-based survey. *International Quarterly of Community Health Education, 20,* 39–58.

Carver, C. S., & Scheier, M. F. (2001). Optimism, pessimism, and self-regulation. In E. C. Chang (Ed.), *Optimism and pessimism: Implications for theory, research, and practice* (pp. 31–51). Washington DC: American Psychological Association.

Carver, C. S., & Scheier, M. F. (2002). Optimism. In C. R. Snyder, & S. J. Lopez (Eds.), *Handbook of positive psychology* (pp. 231–243). Oxford: Oxford University Press.

Carver, C. S., & Scheier, M. F. (2003). Three human strengths. In L. G. Aspinwall, & U. M. Staudinger (Eds.), *A psychology of human strengths: Fundamental questions and future directions for a positive psychology* (87–102). Washington DC: American Psychological Association.

Chang, E. C. (2001). Cultural influences on optimism and pessimism: Differences in western and eastern construals of the self. In E. C. Chang (Ed.), *Optimism and pessimism: Implications for theory, research, and practice* (pp. 257–280). Washington DC: American Psychological Association.

Csikszentmihalyi, M. (1990). *Flow: The psychology of optimal experience.* New York: Harper & Row.

Dickson, J. M., & MacLeod, A. K. (2004). Approach and avoidance goals and plans: Their relationship to anxiety and depression. *Cognitive Therapy and Research, 28,* 415–432.

Emmons, R. A. (2003). Personal goals, life meaning, and virtue: Wellsprings of a positive life. In C. L. M. Keyes, & J. Haidt (Eds.), *Flourishing: Positive psychology and the life well-lived* (pp. 105–123). Washington DC: American Psychological Association.

Frydenberg, E. (2002). Beyond coping: Some paradigms to consider. In E. Frydenberg (Ed.), *Beyond coping: Meeting goals, visions, and challenges* (pp. 3–16). Oxford: Oxford University Press.

Garber, J. (2000). Optimism: Definitions and origins. In J. E. Gilham (Ed.), *The science of optimism and hope* (pp. 299–314). Philadelphia: Templeton Foundation Press.

Gillham, J. E., Shatte, A. J., Reivich, K. J., & Seligman, M. E. P. (2001). Optimism, pessimism, and explanatory style. In E. C. Chang (Ed.), *Optimism and pessimism: Implications for theory, research, and practice* (pp. 53–75). Washington DC: American Psychological Association.

Griffith, B. A., & Graham, C. C. (2004). Meeting needs and making meaning: The pursuit of goals. *Journal of Individual Psychology, 60,* 25–41.

King, I. M. (1987). King's theory of goal attainment. In R. R. Parse (Ed.), *Nursing science: Major paradigms, theories, and critiques* (pp. 107–113). Philadelphia: WB Saunders.

King, I. M. (1989). King's general systems framework and theory. In J. P. Riehl-Sica (Ed.), *Conceptual models for nursing practice* (pp. 149–158). Norwalk, CT: Appleton & Lange.

King, I. M. (1995). The theory of goal attainment. In M. A. Frey & C. L. Sieloff (Eds.), *Advancing King's systems framework and theory of nursing* (pp. 23–32). Thousand Oaks, CA: Sage.

Locke, E. A. (2003). Setting goals for life and happiness. In C. R. Snyder, & S. J. Lopez (Eds.), *Handbook of positive psychology* (pp. 299–312). Oxford: Oxford University Press.

Lopez, S. J., Floyd, R. K., Ulvan, J. C., & Snyder, C. R. (2000). Hope therapy: Helping clients build a house of hope. In C. R. Snyder (Ed.), *Handbook of hope: Theory, measures and applications* (pp. 123–150). San Diego, CA: Academic Press.

Magaletta, P. R., & Oliver, J. M. (1999). The hope construct, will and ways: Their relations with self-efficiency, optimism, and general well-being. *Journal of Clinical Psychology, 55,* 539–551.

Mulkana, S. S., & Hailey, B. J. (2001). The role of optimism in health-enhancing behavior. *American Journal of Health Behavior, 25,* 388–395.

Nakamura, J., & Csikszentmihalyi, M. (2003), The construction of meaning through vital engagement. In C. L. M. Keyes, & J. Haidt (Eds.), *Flourishing: Positive psychology and the life well-lived* (pp. 83–104). Washington DC: American Psychological Association.

Peterson, C. (2000). Optimistic explanatory style and health. In J. E. Gilham (Ed.), *The science of optimism and hope* (pp. 145–161). Philadelphia: Templeton Foundation Press.

Peterson, C., & Bossio, L. H. (2001). Optimism and physical well-being. In E. C. Chang (Ed.), *Optimism and pessimism: Implications for theory, research, and practice* (pp. 127–145). Washington DC: American Psychological Association.

Peterson, C., & Chang, E. C. (2001). Optimism and flourishing. In C. L. M. Keyes, & J. Haidt (Eds.), *Flourishing: Positive psychology and the life well-lived* (pp. 55–79). Washington DC: American Psychological Association.

Pretzer, J. L., & Walsh, C. A. (2001). Optimism, pessimism, and psychotherapy: Implications for clinical practice. In E. C. Chang (Ed.), *Optimism and pessimism: Implications for theory, research, and practice* (pp. 321–346). Washington DC: American Psychological Association.

Reivich, L. V., & Gillham, J. (2003). Learned optimism: The measurement of explanatory style. In S. J. Lopez, & C. R. Snyder (Eds.), *Positive psychological assessment: A handbook of models and measures* (pp. 57–74). Washington DC: American Psychological Association.

Riskind, J. H., Sarampote, C. S., & Mercier, M. A. (1996). For every malady a sovereign cure: Optimism training. *Journal of Cognitive Psychotherapy, 10,* 105–117.

Ryan, R. M., & Deci, E. L. (2000). Self-determination theory and the facilitation of intrinsic motivation, social development, and well-being. *American Psychologist, 55,* 68–78.

Ryff, C. D., & Singer, B. (1998). The role of purpose in life and personal growth in positive human health. In P. T. P. Wong, & P. S. Fry (Eds.), *The human quest for meaning* (pp. 213–225). Mahwah, NJ: Lawrence Erlbaum.

Scheier M. F., & Carver, C. S. (2003). Goals and confidence as self-regulatory elements underlying health and illness behavior. In L. D. Cameron, & H. Leventhal (Eds.), *The self-regulation of health and illness behavior* (pp. 17–41). London: Routledge.

Scheier, M. F., Carver, C. S., & Bridges, M. W. (2002). Optimism, pessimism and psychological well-being. In E. C. Chang (Ed.), *Optimism and pessimism: Implications for theory, research, and practice* (pp. 189–216). Washington DC: American Psychological Association.

Schmuck, P., & Sheldon, K. M. (2001). Life goals and well-being: To the frontiers of life goal research. In P. Schmuck & K. M. Sheldon. *Life goals and well-being: Towards a positive psychology of human striving* (pp. 1–17). Seattle, WA: Hogrefe & Huber.

Schwarzer, R., & Knoll, N. (2003). Positive copying: Mastering demands and searching for meaning. In S. J. Lopez, & C. R. Snyder (Eds.), *Positive psychological assessment: A handbook of models and measures* (pp. 393–409). Washington DC: American Psychological Association.

Sheldon, K. M. (2001). The self-concordance model of healthy goal striving: When personal goals correctly represent the person. In P. Schmuck & K. M. Sheldon (Eds.), *Life goals and well-being: Towards a positive psychology of human striving* (pp. 18–36). Seattle, WA: Hogrefe & Huber.

Wrosch, C., & Scheier, M. F. (2003). Personality and quality of life: The importance of optimism and goal adjustment. *Quality of life research, 12* (Suppl 1), 59–72.

CHAPTER 5

Connections

Concepts
Religion/Spirituality
Social Support

Models and Theories
Watson's Theory of Human Science and
    Human Caring
Attachment Theory
The Belongingness Hypothesis
Intimacy Theory
Physiological Mechanisms
Theory of Human Relatedness

Helpful Lists
Watson's Carative Factors, pg. 66
Attachment Styles, pgs. 66–67
Approaches to Spirituality, pg. 69
Social Support Assessment, pg. 72
Social Activity and Relatedness, pg. 75
Individuality and Goals, pg. 75
Considerations in Nursing Interventions
    to Foster Connectedness, pg. 76

Thought Questions:
1. How do connectedness and relatedness differ?
2. How might reciprocity, mutuality, and synchrony affect nurse-client relationships?
3. Which approach(s) to spirituality affect your life? How do they influence your nursing practice?
4. Can nurses provide social support? If so, how? How can you foster social support by others?
5. How do cultural differences affect perceptions of connection? What are the implications for your nursing practice?
6. What nursing interventions can you provide to promote client perceptions of connectedness?

Chapter Synopsis
This chapter introduces the strength of human connectedness as a resource for health. Connectedness (or connections), are strongly related to meaning, goals, control, capability, confidence, and choice concepts in the Healthiness Theory. The related concepts of spirituality/religion and social support are discussed. Multiple human strength theories such as Watson's theory of human science and human care, attachment theory, the belongingness hypothesis, intimacy theory, physiological mechanisms, and the theory of human relatedness are described. The importance of multicultural competency is

stressed, through discussion of African American, Asian American, Latin American, Native American, and Japanese cultural values related to connectedness. Finally, several intervention strategies to foster connectedness are discussed.

CONNECTEDNESS

Connectedness promotes a sense of comfort and well-being, supports a sense of meaning in life, and reduces anxiety. Connectedness occurs when one individual is actively involved with another individual (interpersonal), object, group (social), or environment (natural or man-made) (Hagerty, Lynch-Sauer, Patusky, and Bouwsema, 1993). Connectedness is a result of an interdependent and interrelated relationship and is part of the "respectful, responsible, trusting, and spiritual operative intention between nurse and client" (Lowe, 2002, p. 6).

Connection and relatedness are often used interchangeably. Relatedness refers to an individual's involvement with other individuals, groups, or the natural environment (Patusky, 2002). It includes feeling cared for, as expressed in liking and concern, and is critical to feeling comfortable and secure, and for self-expression and responsiveness in a relationship (Reis, 2001). Relatedness expresses an individual's worldview beyond the sense of self, and involves connection and commitment to an outside entity (other humans or a spiritual being) or the environment (natural, physical, or social) (Hanley & Abell, 2002). Creative and artistic expressions are inherently relational as are interactions with the natural world and spiritual forces. Mutual relationships are fulfilling and lead to the successful development of personal talents and abilities (self-actualization).

Interaction is a single social event that occurs between individuals, whereas involvement requires the dedication of time or resources within a relationship (Ryan & Solky, 1996) and usually reflects validation. Validation refers to "appreciation for an individual's dispositions, beliefs, or life circumstances. Validation contributes to intimacy and meaningful interaction by suggesting that the other (individual) values and respects the emotional core of the self" (Reis, 2001, p. 80). A shared base of understanding ("getting the facts straight") helps relatedness.

Autonomy support is an important concept concerning relatedness in cultures that emphasize the individual. The need for autonomy refers to the desire to determine personal behavior, take action, and be self-expressive and spontaneous. Autonomy support refers to the ability to understand another's perspective and to encourage their self-expression and action. Typically, autonomy support involves genuinely acknowledging another individual's perceptions, accepting their feelings, and not attempting to control their experience and behavior (Ryan & Solky, 1996). Autonomy support encourages the development, expression, and integration of the self and buffers individuals from negative outcomes during stress. The outcomes of autonomy support include increased self-esteem, self-confidence, feelings of capability and competence, vitality, and feelings of connectedness with others. Autonomy support is needed for social contacts to enhance psychological well-being (Ryan & Solky, 1996).

Patusky (2002) describes a nested ecological approach consisting of four levels of relatedness: the macro system (societal beliefs); ecosystem (groups that affect the immediate setting, e.g., work); microsystem (family unit); and ontogenetic (individual development), all of which provide opportunities for nursing involvement. Within each level, four states of relatedness were identified: connectedness (comfortable involvement), disconnectedness, parallelism, and enmeshment. Competencies that are associated with these states include synchrony, sense of belonging, reciprocity, and mutuality (Patusky, 2002). This theory is discussed more fully in the theory section of this chapter.

A relationship is an ongoing connection between two individuals in which there is a sense of history and some awareness of the nature of the relationship; the participants influence each other's thoughts, feelings and behavior; and they expect to interact again in the future (Reis, 2001). Relationships that heal, soothe, foster growth, facilitate health, and provide satisfaction are essential to a sense of well-being (Ryan & Solky, 1996). The nurse can use the capacity for authentic interaction to draw out and support a client's real feelings, sensibilities, and choices, while providing a sense of support and nurturance (Ryan & Solky, 1996). Consequently, a sense of belonging is experienced when an individual perceives a "fit" with another individual, group, or environment, and feels valued, needed, and important within relationships (Hagerty & Patusky, 2003).

Relationships impact three domains, the affective, the cognitive, and the behavioral. In the *affective* domain the question is: how do people *feel* about each other? In the *cognitive* domain the question is: what thoughts do people *think* about each other? And, in the *behavioral* domain the question is: how do people *treat* each other? (Kenny, 1994). Relationships may also be situational or contextual. The nurse can gain insight into a client's relationships and support base by asking questions related to each domain.

Affirmative interactions are associated with the affective domain. Some qualities of this domain include self-expression to significant others; feeling securely connected to and able to rely on others during stressful circumstances; being responsive and supportive to partners and open to their expressions of need; perceiving with reasonable accuracy a close partner's understanding, valuing, and caring; experiencing genuine enjoyment during interaction with significant others; and coping constructively with negative emotions and interpersonal conflict. When needs are frustrated in a relationship it often triggers harmful negative emotions, maladaptive thinking and behavior, and destructive psychophysiological reactions (Reis, 2001). "Feedback that is perceived as misinformed or irrelevant or that ignores a person's self-understanding, no matter how favorable, is likely to be discounted" (Reis, 2001, p. 80). It has also been shown that task-focused interaction does not increase relatedness.

Relationships are perhaps the most important source of life satisfaction and emotional well-being. Individuals mention close relationships more than anything else when describing what gives life meaning. Men rely on women for their intimacy, while women are more physiologically reactive to negative aspects of social relationships (Ryff & Singer, 2001). Social connections and social support are important for health, recovery from illness, and physiological functioning. For example, conflict and hostility are associated with down-regulation of the immune system (Reis & Gable, 2003), and mortality from all causes is greater among individuals with relatively low levels of social support (Cohen & Wills, 1985; Uchino, Cacioppo, and Kiecolt-Glaser, 1996).

THEORIES

Watson's Human Science and Human Care Theory

Watson's nursing theory is based on her conception of "transpersonal caring" as "a moral ideal of nursing with a concern for preservation of humanity, dignity, and freedom of self" (Watson, 1985, p. 74). Watson wants nursing to concern itself more with meaning, relationships, contexts, and patterns" (p. 2).

Watson identified ten "carative factors," or nursing interventions that she feels are the basis for practice when used with a knowledge base and clinical competence. The carative factors are (Watson, 1989, pp. 227–228):

1. Formation of a humanistic-altruistic system of values.
2. Nurturing of faith and hope.
3. Cultivation of sensitivity to one's self and others.
4. Development of a helping-trusting, human caring relationship.
5. Promotion and acceptance of the expression of positive and negative feelings.
6. Use of creative problem-solving caring processes.
7. Promotion of transpersonal teaching-learning.
8. Provision for a supportive, protective, or corrective mental, physical, sociocultural, and spiritual environment.
9. Assistance with gratification of human needs.
10. Allowance for existential-phenomenologic-spiritual forces.

Watson believes that "connectedness with other, and yet beyond self and other, keeps alive our common humanity" (Watson, 1996, p. 148). The emphasis for nursing is on "helping other(s), through advanced nursing caring-healing modalities, to gain more self-knowledge, self-control, and even self-healing potential" (Watson, 1996, p. 148). This theory fits seamlessly with the philosophy underlying this book.

Attachment Theory

As originally postulated by Bowlby (1969), attachment is an emotional regulation-based control system designed to maintain closeness between infants and caregivers. Its central premise is that infants kept in close proximity with adult caregivers are more likely to survive into adulthood when the infants display appropriate protest behaviors when separated or threatened, and their caregivers respond appropriately to the protests. Ideally the bond between infant and caregiver is secure, so that the infant's expressions of anxiety and distress usually results in sensitive responses from the caregiver. Thus, the developing child feels safe in using the caregiver as a secure base from which to explore the environment. When early caregiving is consistent and responsive, the child feels secure, internalizes being worthy of love, and comes to view others (besides the caregiver) as sources of support, comfort, and affection (Reis, 2001). However, three attachment styles have been proposed (Reis, 2001):

1. *Avoidance*—an insecure style characterized by avoiding intimacy and closeness and feeling uncomfortable with relying on others for support.

2. *Preoccupation*—an ambivalent, insecure style characterized by anxiety about social relationships and being preoccupied with establishing and maintaining closeness.
3. *Secure*—is characterized by a comfortable balance between preoccupation and distance, and close relationships are perceived as a source of pleasure and satisfaction.

Insecure attachment occurs when a caregiver's response is chronically inadequate or poorly matched to the infant's needs. One form of insecurity, avoidance, is thought to result from inattentive or emotionally cold responses to the infant's distress and desire for comfort. Avoidance involves learning to cope with anxiety through emotional distancing and self-reliance. Preoccupation, originally called anxious-ambivalence, is thought to result from inconsistent caregiving, which may be intrusive one moment and unresponsive the next. Individuals dealing with this type of insecurity are prone to anxiety and other negative emotions. They are often preoccupied with and dependent on close relationships, but are also vigilant in looking for signs of acceptance and rejection and are thus easily angered and disillusioned. "At its core, then, attachment is a theory about how individuals experience the emotions of love, fear, anger, jealousy, sadness, disappointment, anxiety, loneliness, and contentment in the context of their close relationships" (Reis, 2001, pp. 62–63).

The Belongingness Hypothesis

Individuals naturally need to establish and sustain belongingness through frequent, positive interactions with a few other individuals within the context of long-term, stable, caring relationships. To satisfy the need to belong, individuals must believe that others care about their welfare and like (or love) them. A change in belongingness (i.e., death or broken relationship) results in strong and pervasive emotions, although the loss of a relationship with one individual can to some extent be replaced by another (Baumeister & Leary, 1995).

Intimacy Theory

Intimacy is interactive and begins when one individual expresses personal thoughts, feelings, and information to another. The self-expression may be verbal or nonverbal, implicit or explicit, semantic or behavioral. All that matters is that the revealed content pertains to the emotional core of the self. The next step depends on the partner's reaction. Responses that are supportive and accepting help develop intimacy, but inappropriate, disinterested, or rejecting responses thwart intimacy. Responses that contribute to the perception that an individual is understood, validated, and cared for by a partner are most likely to foster intimacy (Reis, 2001).

Intimacy theory (Reis & Patrick, 1996; Reis & Shaver, 1988) is derived in part from attachment theory. It is proposed that emotionally close adult relationships fulfill many of the same functions as attachment relationships do in childhood. This model portrays intimacy as an interactive process with three components: an individual's expression of thoughts and feelings through verbal, nonverbal, and behavioral channels; the partner's response, in terms of appropriateness and supportiveness; and the individual's perception of the partner's response. Intimacy is experienced when the sequence of expression and response leads to feeling understood, validated, and cared for. Most intimate relationships are mutual and reciprocated, with partners typically alternating between expression and response (Reis, 2001).

Intimacy theory implies that the most emotionally important interactions are those in which significant self-disclosure occurs with a responsive partner. What matters most is how responsive the partner is to the individual's core psychological self, not the details of self-disclosure or the actual response. Thus, positive emotions such as love, happiness, and acceptance, and negative emotions such as sadness, anger, and loneliness, can be described as reactions to a partner's response. Because they are more likely to involve emotionally self-relevant exchanges, interactions that involve intimate partners should be more important to emotional well-being than interactions that involve less close partners (Reis, 2001).

Physiological Mechanisms

Uchino, Cacioppo and Kiecolt-Glaser (1996) indicate that social relationships have as strong an impact on health as the known standard risk factors of smoking, hypertension, and inactivity. Social relationships can positively affect health by providing (a) stress-buffering effects; (b) familial sources of support; and (c) emotional support. Emotional support has been found to be a more persistent predictor of neuroendocrine function than informational support, social ties (e.g., integration), instrumental support, or negative aspects of social relationships (Berkman, 1995). It is known that social relationships influence aspects of immune function, especially cellular immunity and natural killer cell activity (Berkman, 1995). Increased social support is associated with better cardiovascular regulation (Uchino et al., 1996) and may be important in reducing cardiovascular reactivity to psychosocial stressors. Social support and interactions have been linked to multiple indicators such as: "heart rate, blood pressure, cholesterol, epinephrine, norepinephrine, [and] autonomic activation (free fatty acids and galvanic skin response)" (Ryff & Singer, 2001, p. 14).

Theory of Human Relatedness

Relatedness is defined as "an individual's level of involvement with persons, objects, groups or natural environments and the concurrent level of comfort or discomfort associated with that involvement" (Hagerty et al., 1993, p. 292). Relatedness focuses on an individual's perception of the quality of relationship with other individuals, objects, environments, society, or the self. Relatedness may be instrumental, with an emphasis on tasks and goals rather than on the relationship, or expressive, with an emphasis on the sharing of meaningful feelings including warmth and affection.

Different states of relatedness may include connectedness, disconnectedness (lack of relatedness), parallelism (communication that is concurrent but not connected), and enmeshment (too close an involvement). Contributing to relatedness are social processes such as sense of belonging (feeling an integral part of the system), reciprocity, mutuality, and synchrony (Hagerty et al., 1993). Relatedness is communicated through feelings of trust, comfort, meaningfulness and connection.

Reciprocity is defined as "the individual's perception of an equitable, alternating, inter-change with another person, object, or environment." (Hagerty & Patusky, 2003, p. 148). Mutuality is the real or symbolic perception of shared visions, goals, sentiments, or char-acteristics, and shared acceptance of differences. Synchrony is the experience of being in harmony with internal rhythms in space-time or through external interactions. Each interaction is an opportunity for connection and goal achievement.

RELATED CONCEPTS

Religion/Spirituality

Spirituality refers to an intrinsic, transcendent quality of discovering meaning in a rela-tionship with a supernatural being and is a prerequisite to authentic religiousness.

Three approaches to spirituality have been identified:

1. *Transcendent approach*—stresses a relational aspect to God; faith in God or a supreme being; feeling a connectedness or oneness with God; integration of all human dimensions; harmonious interconnectedness; and capacity for inner knowing, inner strength, and the freedom and creativity of self-determination.
2. *Value guidance*—stresses self-potential, gives meaning and purpose to life, and intrapersonal transcendence (a source of authority that integrates all the body dimensions).
3. *Structuralist-behaviorist*—stresses religious commitment and religiosity.

Spirituality motivates, enables, empowers, and provides hope. "Giving and receiving love and forgiveness from others, and developing relationships of trust and mutuality can promote hope and inner strength" (Coyle, 2002, p. 595). Elements of spirituality include balance, fostering community, seeking to uncover rather than create, nurturing and sup-port, feeling respected, belonging, growth, and personal transformation, learning, and caring. Nurses who have a deeper sense of their own spirituality are better equipped to deal with the spiritual situations of others. As part of a health assessment, nurses should ask clients about their perceptions of spirituality and then should seek ways to respect and honor those perceptions in providing care. It is the journey, not the achievement of the vision that should be emphasized (Pesut, 2003).

In contrast, religion addresses "the personal beliefs, values, and activities pertinent to that which is supernatural, mysterious and awesome, which transcends immediate situa-tions and which pertains to questions of final causes and ultimate ends of man and the universe" (Moberg, 1970, p. 175). All religions include beliefs in a supernatural intelligent being or beings; a worldview that interprets the significance of human life; belief in expe-rience after death; a moral code believed to be sanctioned by a supernatural being; prayer and ritual, sacred objects and places; and mystical, awesome religious experiences.

Wong (1998) has identified three aspects of religion: an extrinsic dimension charac-terized by institutional or organized religious activity; an intrinsic dimension character-ized by sincere and devout commitment to religious beliefs; and a quest dimension characterized by open-ended readiness to confront existential questions.

In a qualitative study with 12 subjects, Fletcher (2004) found that religious beliefs could divide the sample into three groups: the believers, the belongers, and the doubters.

The "believers" in a strong religious truth found meaning through a relationship with a Supreme Being and trust in the Bible rather than through social relationships. In contrast, the "belongers" and the "doubters," whose belief systems were more fluid in personal interpretation and relativism, needed positive social interaction and reinforcement within the religious community.

Religion may bring a sense of coherence, hope, and significance to life, helping individuals rise above everyday frustrations. By putting death into perspective, religion provides both direction and support to life (Wong, 1998). The shared system of religious rituals and symbols also provides a sense of community. Many researchers have reported a positive relationship between religious involvement and mental or physical health, which tends to increase as people grow older (Wong, 1998).

Social Support

Social relations involve the many factors and interpersonal interactions that characterize social exchanges without revealing the nature, content, or quality of relationships (Antonucci, 2001). Social support refers to the actual exchange of support, "an interpersonal transaction involving…aid, affect, or affirmation" (Antonucci, 2001, p. 429). Social support promotes health when it provides a sense of belonging and intimacy, and helps individuals to be more capable (Berkman, 1995).

When individuals feel valued, competent, worthy, and capable as a result of social relations, they feel socially supported. Perceived (subjective) social support is a trait-like sense of acceptance that is highly related to health and well-being, especially when it matches specific needs required by an individual (McNally & Newman, 1999). Self-esteem is the best predictor of perceived support. In contrast, enacted (objective) social support can be measured by the amount of time spent or the number of contacts made with an individual. Measures of perceived and enacted support do not appear to be strongly related (Lakey & Lutz, 1996), indicating separate concepts.

Structural measures of support assess the existence and interconnections between various social relationships, whereas functional measures assess the particular support functions that social relationships serve (e.g., emotional or informational support). Situation-specific social support is tied to coping with a particular stressful event. And, support reciprocity views support as a loan or indebtedness being repaid for an earlier provision of support. "Large-scale macro social, economic, and welfare policies influence the ability of families and communities to maintain high levels of [enacted] social integration and support" (Berkman, 1995, p. 251).

Social support may be emotional, informational, social, or instrumental. Emotional or esteem support is information that makes an individual feel esteemed and accepted. Emotional support may include expressions of concern and caring including talking, listening, and touching. The nurse can enhance a client's self-esteem by appreciating their individual worth and experiences and accepting the client despite any difficulties or personal faults (Cohen & Wills, 1985). Informational support can be provided by helping the client to define, understand, and cope with problems. Social companionship is spending time with others in leisure and recreational activities, and instrumental support is the provision of tangible financial aid, material resources, and needed services. "Social support may have beneficial effects through social (e.g., stress-buffering), psychological (e.g., affective states), and behavioral (e.g., health-promoting) mechanisms" (Uchino et al., 1996, p. 502). The negative aspects of social relationships are independent of the positive aspects of support.

Components of social support include support schema, supportive relationships, and support transactions. Support schemas are perceptions about the availability of others. These perceptions tend to be stable across time and situations, and are the strongest predictors of personal adjustment. Because support schemas are positively related to self-appraisals, they tend to be more effective in developing supportive relationships in new social environments. They are also more interpersonally sensitive and more strongly desired as potential sources of social support, and have short-term and long-term consequences. Supportive relationships, in turn, provide emotional support, tangible assistance, cognitive information, and directive guidance.

Supportive transactions can be explicit requests for assistance, or indirect communication expressing need without actually asking for assistance. The interpersonal context strongly influences the recipient's appraisals of potentially supportive behavior (Pierce, Sarason, Sarason, Joseph, and Henderson, 1996). For example, a simple request of "can I help you" when another individual seems to be having difficulty crossing the street can be a supportive transaction.

In stressful situations "the buffering model suggests that 'support buffers' protect individuals from the potentially pathogenic influence of stressful events. The alternative model proposes that social resources have a beneficial effect irrespective of whether persons are under stress" (Cohen & Wills, 1985, p. 310). Both models contribute to understanding the relationships between social support and health. Social networks can provide regular positive experiences, a set of stable socially rewarded roles in the community, a sense of predictability and stability in life, a recognition of self-worth, and may be related to health outcomes through emotionally induced effects on neuroendocrine or immune system functioning (Cohen & Wills, 1985).

Support may reduce or prevent a stress appraisal response between the stressful event (or expectation of that event) and a stress reaction. By reducing or eliminating the stress reaction or by directly influencing physiological processes, adequate support may mediate the experience of stress and the onset of pathology. For example, nursing support may alleviate the impact of stress appraisal by (a) providing a solution to the problem; (b) reducing the perceived importance of the problem; (c) tranquilizing the neuro-endocrine system to reduce reactivity to perceived stress (e.g., providing medication); or (d) facilitating healthful behaviors (Cohen & Wills, 1985).

More positive (and fewer negative) social ties to a spouse, other family members, and friends have been associated with significantly lower levels of symptoms, fewer chronic conditions, and higher subjective health for members of both genders (Ryff & Singer, 2001). Close relationships may be a particularly important source of social support. The ability to buffer stress requires a reasonable match between the coping requirements and the perceived adequacy of available support (Cohen & Wills, 1985). Thus, social support is more effective when it closely matches the demands of a particular situation. Anxiety in preparation for an examination might only require a soothing expression of understanding, while a diagnosis of cancer is best addressed with ongoing support that varies as the context changes.

An initial assessment by the nurse of a client's social support should include:

1. Types of support required
2. Sources of support
3. Reciprocity of support
4. Costs and benefits associated with support
5. Satisfaction with support
6. Underuse and overuse of support resources
7. Appropriate timing and duration of support

MULTICULTURAL COMPETENCY

Culture provides a collective understanding of a shared way of life, and a vocabulary of symbols to express and assign meaning to various aspects of social life (Dilworth-Anderson & Marshall, 1996). In the following section, selected symbols assigned to connectedness (viewed as social support) are described for five different cultures: African Americans, Hispanic Americans, Asian Americans, Native Americans, and the Japanese. It is important for nurses to be aware of the different cultural influences affecting clients and their families. This information helps to understand client reactions, family structures, social support networks, and how the clients see their role within their cultural framework. Having a grasp of these concepts enables nurses to respond with insight and sensitivity to cultures that may be very different than their own.

African Americans

The cultural context in which African Americans give and receive social support in their families has been shaped by the "veil of slavery," where survival became a group effort. Although slavery ended in 1865, African Americans were still restricted from access to health care, education, employment, legal rights, and adequate housing needed to support a family. As a result, the family and church in the African American community provided the social support that was often lacking due to discrimination from enacted laws and accepted practices within American society (Dilworth-Anderson & Marshall, 1996).

Fluid and flexible boundaries in African American families allow the inclusion of dependent generations into existing households. Family support has traditionally included helping with child care, sharing households, and providing emotional support to close and distant kin (Dilworth-Anderson & Marshall, 1996).

Motherhood and parenting among African Americans have very strong traditional cultural meanings, which include mothering within the extended family as opposed to the nuclear family; lack of sex-role segregation in parenting within the family, and motherhood separate from economic dependency on a male breadwinner in the home. Parenting and mothering are roles assumed by others in the family or even individuals outside the family.

Individualization is not necessarily viewed as a developmental task and children are not socialized nor given the opportunity to develop on their own. Instead, family enmeshment is encouraged as the goal of socialization, which fosters a sense of "intergenerational reciprocity, responsibility, and the maintenance of the kin network. For example, the authoritarian parenting style among African Americans encourages children to respect their elders, obey their parents, and be responsible for others…Elderly blacks receive a great deal of support and care-giving from their children," with older women more likely than older men to receive support (Dilworth-Anderson & Marshall, 1996, p. 72–73).

Hispanic Americans

The term Hispanic is used to represent a diverse group of people of Spanish origin who came to this country as free immigrants. Most Hispanics have a family-centered culture that serves as the core of their social support system. These family-centered cultures include a social support system that reflects close and distant kin and the godparents of children in the family (Dilworth-Anderson & Marshall, 1996). Hispanics preserve their customs through family and community rituals, in which mutual obligation and reciprocity are expected. They tend to live in close proximity to one another, share in child-rearing, and speak their native language. Among Cubans, friends in addition to family give and receive social support from one another, but among Mexican Americans it is the family that is a major source of identity, self-worth, and social support (Dilworth-Anderson & Marshall, 1996).

In Hispanic families, the parent-child pair is often considered more important than the marital couple. There is strong support for age and gender hierarchies, with older males generally held in higher esteem than their younger counterparts. Older women, particularly grandmothers, are revered in the culture. "The caretaking of these older women is typically based on a system of intergenerational reciprocity…The care of the elderly includes providing material and emotional support" (Dilworth-Anderson & Marshall, 1996, p. 73–74).

Asian Americans

Although very diverse, Asian Americans share a common thread of family-centered social support systems. These support systems are maintained through a cultural sense of family loyalty and the predominance of group over individual concerns (Dilworth-Anderson & Marshall, 1996). Asian American families tend to maintain strict hierarchies based on gender, and respect and honor older individuals, especially parents. These hierarchies are reinforced by a strong sense of shame when obligations and societal expectations are not met. Multiple generations typically live close to one another. Lifestyles that are moderate in behavior, self-discipline, modesty, and patience are valued as they contribute to harmony (Dilworth-Anderson & Marshall, 1996).

The care of Asian American children demonstrates the values of family harmony versus individual needs, self-control, and ancestor worship (Dilworth-Anderson & Marshall, 1996). Individual achievements are highly valued and are not a source of envy because they bring honor to the entire family. The social support context is characterized by discipline, self-control, and extended family networks (Dilworth-Anderson & Marshall, 1996).

In a comparative study of immigrant Chinese and European American values, Rothbaum, Morelli, Pott, and Liu-Constant (2000) found that closeness is characterized by an overarching theme of harmony in immigrant Chinese families and by an overarching theme of romance in European American families. Physical closeness is defined as "aspects of physicality that deal with the boundary between the self's and others' bodies" (Rothbaum et al., 2000, p. 334). Consistent with other Asian American cultures, immigrant Chinese parents emphasize the family unit, and place greater importance on inhibition of expression, adherence to correct values, and hierarchy of relations. European Americans, in contrast, emphasize psychological benefits of physical closeness and the child's expression of wants and feelings, more often view independence as celebrating the child's distinctiveness, and place greater importance on the intimacy, pleasure, and exclusiveness of the married couple (Rothbaum et al., 2000). European Americans express patterns of feelings of warmth, a sense of self-esteem, feelings of intimacy, and feelings of enjoyment and pleasure associated with physical closeness. In contrast, immigrant Chinese express a sense of family connection, feelings of being safe and comfortable, a sense that love is reciprocated, and feelings of respect as well as love.

Native Americans

Emotional, material, and instrumental support is associated with Native American extended family relational networks that foster strong interrelationships and a mutual assistance network (Dilworth-Anderson & Marshall, 1996). However, in contrast to Asian American families, the kin network of Native American families encourages the strong value of autonomy in children. The children are seldom punished, are generally allowed freedom in making decisions, and are encouraged to develop self-control within the relational networks in which they live. The rearing of children is guided by both material and spiritual forces. Traditional affiliation with the cultural group, rather than their individual affiliation, provides the framework for social support (Dilworth-Anderson & Marshall, 1996). In this culture the sense of time is present oriented, rhythmic, and cyclic rather than linear.

In Native American culture, support of the elderly is fostered by the values of the importance of the group, a sense of individual autonomy, and lack of competition. "The elderly are given important tribal roles, are respected by younger generations, and receive and give intergenerational caregiving, and many live in extended family households" (Dilworth-Anderson & Marshall, 1996, p. 75–76). Support and care to the elderly is often provided using community-based and in-home services (because of distrust of the government) provided by the extended kin system, which includes spouses, adult children, and grandchildren. Family and group needs and desires take precedence over those of the individual (Lowe, 2002).

Japanese Culture

Amae, the indigenous Japanese concept of relatedness, places an implicit emphasis on psychological dependence. Amae involves an indulgent dependency that includes being accepted for asking for something that individuals are perfectly capable of doing for themselves, some expectation of being understood and accepted, and the presumption that others will be indulgent and accepting (Behrens, 2004). These expectations may be perfectly understandable within the family, but nurses raised in Western cultures expect clients to do as much for themselves as possible. These differences of expectations can lead to misunderstandings and conflict between the client and nurse. Five categories of Amae are described as: affective (based on emotions), manipulative (where one individual takes advantage of the other), reciprocal (mutual), obligatory (based on a sense of debt), and presumptive (based on assumptions). The pattern of attachment represents the quality of the relationship; the quantity of amae is measurable.

INTERVENTIONS

How can a nurse best use each interaction in a therapeutic way in a limited time? It is important for nurses to identify their own needs for relatedness and feeling close and connected to significant others, without transferring that need inappropriately to client relationships (Reis, Sheldon, Gable, Roscoe, and Ryan, 2000). For example, a client cannot be a friend of the nurse. The human tendency to form strong, stable interpersonal bonds is referred to as the "need to belong." Reis and colleagues (2000) have identified seven types of social activity that might contribute to a sense of relatedness:

1. Communicating personally relevant matters within a context of shared commonalities
2. Participating in shared activities
3. Spending informal social time with a group of friends
4. Feeling understood and appreciated
5. Participating in pleasant or enjoyable activities
6. Avoiding arguments and conflict that create distance and feelings of disengagement with significant others
7. Avoiding self-conscious or insecure feelings that direct attention toward the self and away from others

Hagerty and Patusky (2003) stress that in the current environment of short-term nurse-client relationships, the emphasis should be placed on the client's achievement of individuality and mutually set goals. Some specific considerations include:

1. Addressing client's expectations directly, through cognitive restructuring
2. Preparing clients to encounter negative thinking from others
3. Focusing on being rather than doing within a context of exchange and sharing
4. Validating clients' experiences while fostering hope
5. Acknowledging reciprocity, equity, and the give and take of relationships and perspectives
6. Identifying shared commonalities that validate the client using presence, exchange, unconditionality, respect, trust, partnership, and silence
7. Balancing interdependence and interrelatedness

Specific social support interventions that nurses can use include: cognitive therapy strategies such as correcting distorted thinking that may be related to distressed mood (gather information); training in social skills (initiate conversation, facilitate dialogue, foster ability to talk about interests, increase self-disclosure, encourage expression of positive emotion); and reflective journaling. In a study with cancer clients, Pierce and colleagues (1996) found that the following considerations were important in fostering connectedness:

1. Physical presence
2. Expressions of concern
3. Calm acceptance
4. Expression of optimism
5. Provision of useful information or advice
6. Expression of special understanding because of similar experience
7. Provision of technically competent care
8. Being pleasant and kind

However, "studies designed to increase perceived social support have not provided strong evidence that social support can be improved very easily" (Lakey & Lutz, 1996, p. 446). Because the nurse can personally provide only limited social support, the client's ability to garner support from others should be encouraged.

References
Antonucci, T. C. (2001). An examination of social networks, social support and sense of control. In J. E. Birren & K. W. Schaie (Eds.), *Handbook of the psychology of aging* (5th ed., pp. 427–453). San Diego, CA: Academic Press.

Baumeister, R. F., & Leary, M. R. (1995). The need to belong: Desire for interpersonal attachments as a fundamental human motivation. *Psychological Bulletin, 117,* 497–529.

Behrens, K. Y. (2004). A multifaceted view of the concept of Amae: Reconsidering the indigenous Japanese concept of relatedness. *Human Development, 47,* 1–27.

Berkman, L. F. (1995). The role of social relations in health promotion. *Psychosomatic Medicine, 57,* 245–254.

Bowlby, J. (1969). *Attachment and loss* (Vol. 1, Attachment). New York: Basic Books.

Cohen, S., & Wills, T. A. (1985). Stress, social support, and the buffering hypothesis. *Psychological Bulletin, 98,* 310–357.

Coyle, J. (2002). Spirituality and health: Towards a framework for exploring the relationship between spirituality and health. *Journal of Advanced Nursing, 37,* 589–597.

Dilworth-Anderson, P., & Marshall, S. (1996). Social support in its cultural context. In G. R. Pierce, B. R. Sarason, & I. G. Sarason (Eds.), *Handbook of social support and the family* (pp. 67–79). New York: The Plenum Press.

Fletcher, S. K. (2004). Religion and life meaning: Differentiating between religious beliefs and religious community in constructing life meaning. *Journal of Aging Studies, 18,* 171–185.

Hagerty, B. M., & Patusky, K. L. (2003). Reconceptualizing the nurse-patient relationship. *Journal of Nursing Scholarship, 35,* 145–150.

Hagerty, B. M. K., Lynch-Sauer, J., Patusky, K. L., & Bouwsema, M. (1993). An emerging theory of human relatedness. *Image: Journal of Nursing Scholarship, 25,* 291–296.

Hanley, S. J., & Abell, S. C. (2002). Maslow and relatedness: Creating an interpersonal model of self-actualization. *Journal of Humanistic Psychology, 42,* 37–57.

Kenny, D. A. (1994). Using the social relations model to understand relationships. In R. Erber & R. Gilmour (Eds.), *Theoretical frameworks for personal relationships* (pp. 111–127). Hillsdale, NJ: Lawrence Erlbaum.

Lakey, B., & Lutz, C. J. (1996). Social support and preventive and therapeutic interventions. In G. R.

Pierce, B. R. Sarason, & I. G. Sarason (Eds.), *Handbook of social support and the family* (pp. 435–465). New York: The Plenum Press.

Lowe, J. (2002). Balance and harmony through connectedness: The intentionality of Native American nurses. *Holistic Nursing Practice, 16,* 4–11.

McNally, S. T., & Newman, S. (1999). Objective and subjective conceptualizations of social support. *Journal of Psychosomatic Research, 46,* 309–314.

Moberg, D. C. (1970). Religion in the later years. In A. M. Huffman (Ed.), *The daily needs and interests of older persons* (pp. 175–191). Springfield, IL: Charles C. Thomas.

Patusky, K. L. (2002). Relatedness theory as a framework for the treatment of fatigued women. *Archives of Psychiatric Nursing, XVI,* 224–231.

Pesut, B. (2003). Developing spirituality in the curriculum: Worldviews, intrapersonal connectedness, interpersonal connectedness. *Nursing Education Perspectives, 24,* 290–294.

Pierce, G. R., Sarason, B. R., Sarason, I. G., Joseph, H. J., & Henderson, C. A. (1996). Conceptualizing and assessing social support in the context of the family. In G. R. Pierce, B. R. Sarason, & I. G. Sarason (Eds.), *Handbook of social support and the family* (pp. 3–23). New York: The Plenum Press.

Reis, H. T. (2001). Relationship experiences and emotional well-being. In C. D. Ryff & B. H. Singer (Eds.), *Emotion, social relationships, and health* (pp. 57–86). Oxford: Oxford University Press.

Reis, H. T., & Gable, S. L. (2003). Toward a positive psychology of relationships. In C. L. M. Keyes & S. Haidt (Eds.), *Flourishing: Positive psychology and the life well-lived* (pp. 129–159). Washington DC: American Psychological Association.

Reis, H. T., & Patrick, B. C. (1996). Attachment and intimacy: Component processes. In E. T. Higgins & A. Kruglanski (Eds.), *Social psychology: Handbook of basic principles* (pp. 523–563). New York: Guilford.

Reis, H. T., & Shaver, P. (1988). Intimacy as an interpersonal process. In S. Duck (Ed.), *Handbook of personal relationships* (pp. 367–389). Chichester, UK: Wiley.

Reis, H. T., Sheldon, K. M., Gable, S. L., Roscoe, J., & Ryan, R. M. (2000). Daily well-being: The role of autonomy, competence, and relatedness. *Personality and Social Psychology, 26,* 419–435.

Rothbaum, F., Morelli, G., Pott, M., & Liu-Constant, Y. (2000). Immigrant-Chinese and Euro-American patents' physical closeness with young children: Themes of family relatedness. *Journal of Family Psychology, 14,* 334–348.

Ryan, R. M., & Solky, J. A. (1996). What is supportive about social support? In G. R. Pierce, B. R. Sarason, & I. G. Sarason (Eds.), *Handbook of social support and the family* (pp. 249–267). New York: The Plenum Press.

Ryff, C. D., & Singer, B. H. (2001). Introduction: Integrating emotion into the study of social relationships and health. In C. D. Ryff & B. H. Singer (Eds.), *Emotion, social relationships and health* (pp. 3–22). Oxford: Oxford University Press.

Uchino, B. N., Cacioppo, J. T., & Kiecolt-Glaser, J. K. (1996). The relationship between social support and physiological processes: A review with emphasis on underlying mechanisms and implications for health. *Psychological Bulletin, 119,* 488–531.

Watson, J. (1985). *Nursing: Human science and human care.* Norwalk, CT: Appleton-Century-Crofts.

Watson, J. (1989). Watson's philosophy and theory of human caring in nursing. In J. P. Riehl-Sica (Ed.), *Conceptual models for nursing practice* (pp. 219–235). Norwalk CT: Appleton & Lange.

Watson, J. (1996). Watson's theory of transpersonal caring. In P. H. Walker & B. Neuman (Eds.), *A blueprint for use of nursing models: Education, research, practice and administration* (pp. 141–162). New York: National League for Nursing.

Wong, P. T. P. (1998). Meaning and successful aging. In I. B.Weiner, (Ed.), *The human quest for meaning: A handbook of psychological research and clinical applications* (pp. 359–394). Mahwah, NJ: Lawrence Erlbaum.

CHAPTER 6

Power Part One: Capability

Concepts
Self-Efficacy
Agency
Self-Care Agency
Competence

Models and Theories
Orem's Theory of Self-Care Agency
Self-Determination Theory

Helpful Lists
Orem's Requisites for Self-Care Agency,
    pgs. 80–81
Sources of Information on Self-Efficacy,
    pgs. 82–83

Thought Questions
1. What is capability? How does it differ from self-efficacy, mastery, and competence?
2. How does choice affect perceptions of capability?
3. How is capability experienced by clients from Eastern cultures?
4. How can you as a nurse enhance clients' perceptions of capability?

Chapter Synopsis
This chapter introduces the human strength of capability, a component of power in the Healthiness Theory, as a resource for health. Capability is closely related to the concepts of meaning, goals, choice, connection, confidence, and capacity in the Healthiness Theory. The related concepts of self-efficacy, self-care efficacy, agency, and competence will be differentiated from each other and capability. Orem's theory of self-care agency and the theory of self-determination are discussed. Finally, the important differences are presented between independent and interdependent cultural styles affecting capability beliefs.

CAPABILITY

Capability is the self-perceived belief in the individual's ability to achieve desired goals. Therefore, capability is influenced by the individual's choices, sense of control, and confidence in accomplishing goals. It is similar to the concept of self agency, where individuals see themselves capable of shaping motives, behavior, and future possibilities. However, in contrast to the concept of competence, capability does not indicate skill or proficiency in a task. Capability is a belief not an action.

Capability requires confidence, creativity, and general intellectual and communication abilities. It also calls for specialized knowledge in order to perform in a particular content area. Other, more general abilities include: oral and written mastery of an individual's native language, mathematical knowledge; the ability to read and quickly process written information; media competence; independent learning strategies; social competencies; and divergent thinking, critical judgments, and self-criticism.

In contrast, self-efficacy is an evaluation of the ability to perform a specific task. Bandura (1997) claims that self-efficacy should be assessed at the optimal level of specificity that corresponds to the specific task being assessed and the domain of functioning being analyzed. For example, an individual might have a great deal of self-efficacy about building a table. Thus, according to Bandura, self-efficacy should be assessed at the most appropriate level, in this case building a table, within the specific domain of carpentry. "Self-efficacy is not a personality trait, but a temporary and easy to influence characteristic that is strictly situation- and task-related" (Van der Bijl & Shortridge-Baggett, 2001, p. 190).

THEORIES

Orem's Theory of Self-Care Agency

Orem's nursing theory of self-care agency has been derived from her Theory of Self-Care Deficit. This theory addresses two types of agency: self-care agency and dependent-care agency. Self-care agency is defined as the *capability* to identify what must be controlled or managed in order for adults to regulate their own functioning and development, describe the components (requisites, technologies, and care measures) of their therapeutic self-care, and perform the measures that will meet their self-care requirements. Dependent-care agency addresses the needs of adults who have health-derived or health-associated limitations of self-care agency, which, according to the theory, places them in socially dependent relationships for care (Orem, 1995). Only self-care agency is related to the Healthiness Theory concept of capability.

Ten self-care agency "powers" that enable the performance of actions required for self-care are (Orem, 1995):

1. Maintaining attention and exercising requisite vigilance.
2. Controlling the use of available physical energy necessary for the initiation and continuation of self-care operations.
3. Controlling body movements required for the initiation and completion of self-care operations.
4. Being able to reason within a self-care frame of reference.
5. Having motivation (i.e., goal orientation) for self-care.
6. Making and carrying out decisions about self-care.
7. Acquiring, retaining, and using technical knowledge about self-care from authoritative sources.

8. Having a repertoire of cognitive, perceptual, manipulative, communication, and interpersonal skills for self-care operations.
9. Organizing self-care actions or action systems to achieve regulatory goals of self-care.
10. Being able to consistently perform self-care operations, while integrating them with relevant aspects of personal, family, and community living.

Self-Determination Theory

Self-determination theory (SDT) (see Chapter 4) investigates "people's inherent growth tendencies and innate psychological needs that are the bases for their self-motivation and personality integration, as well as the conditions that foster those positive processes" (Ryan & Deci, 2000, p. 68). This theory considers agency, relatedness, and autonomy as essential requirements for optimal functioning. Authentically motivated individuals are more interested, excited, and confident, which results in enhanced performance, persistence and creativity, heightened vitality, self-esteem, and general well-being (Ryan & Deci, 2000).

Intrinsic motivation is a natural inclination toward assimilation, mastery, spontaneous interest, and exploration, and is demonstrated by learning, seeking out novelty and challenges, and extending and exercising personal capacities (Ryan & Deci, 2000). The theory proposes that intrinsic motivation is enhanced though internally generated feelings of self-agency. These feelings occur in situations where feedback is free from demeaning evaluations, and/or external rewards, and directs individuals toward greater effectiveness.

To enhance intrinsic motivation, feelings of capability must be accompanied by autonomy (Ryan & Deci, 2000). Intrinsic motivation is also aided by a sense of security and relatedness. Nurses can foster autonomy by providing clients with choices, acknowledging their feelings, and supporting opportunities for client self-direction. These actions enhance the client's intrinsic motivation by increasing their feelings of autonomy. Activities that hold intrinsic interest because of novelty, challenge, or aesthetic value also promote intrinsic motivation (Ryan & Deci, 2000). Intrinsic motivation refers to doing an activity for the inherent satisfaction of the activity itself.

Extrinsic motivation involves performing an activity to attain a particular outcome. A subtheory within SDT, known as Organismic Integration Theory (OIT), has been developed by Ryan and Deci (2000). This theory outlines different forms of extrinsic motivation such as external, introjected, identified, and integrated regulation. It also presents the contexts influencing the internalization and integration of factors such as compliance, self-control, personal importance, and self-congruence.

RELATED CONCEPTS

Self-Efficacy

Self-efficacy refers to an individual's perceived ability to perform a specific behavior. Three characteristics of self-efficacy are human agency, personal control, and perceived competence. Bandura's (1986) social cognitive theory assigns a central role to cognitive, vicarious, self-regulatory, and self-reflective processes in adaptation and change. Human functioning is viewed as the result of the reciprocal interplay of personal, behavioral, and environmental influences (Pajares, 2002).

It has been suggested that self-efficacy beliefs provide the foundation for motivation, well-being, and personal accomplishment. These beliefs mediate knowledge and action, influence behavior and the environment in which they occur, and determine the effort and perseverance expended on the behavior (Berarducci & Lengacher, 1998). Self-efficacy is also a critical determinant of self-regulation. Generally, individuals are proactively engaged in their own development and what they believe about themselves is critical in exercising control, choice, challenge, and capability (Pajares, 2002).

Efficacy expectation is the belief that individuals can perform a particular behavior in order to produce a specific outcome. Outcome expectation is the result that is anticipated when the behavior is performed (Bandura, 1994, p. 71). For example, a nurse straightens and tightens a client's bed linens with the expectation of making the client more comfortable. Perceived self-efficacy is defined as "people's beliefs about their capabilities to produce designated levels of performance that exercise influence over events that affect their lives." Another, simpler, definition is that self-efficacy is the "capacity for producing a desired result or effect" (Soukhanov, 1992, p. 622).

Efficacy expectations have several dimensions including magnitude (the degree of difficulty involved in a task), generality (the degree an expectation can be generalized from one situation to another), and strength (the confidence individuals have in mastering a particular task). Motivation, affective states, and actions are believed to be based more on what individuals believe than on what may be objectively true. Consequently, knowing what to do and actually doing it are affected by an individual's belief in being able to perform the behavior. Perceived self-efficacy affects both the effort and determination needed to accomplish a task despite any obstacles. Individuals with high self-efficacy and self-esteem approach difficult tasks with a competitive sense toward mastery (Berarducci & Lengacher, 1998; Van der Bijl & Shortridge-Baggett, 2001). Higher self-efficacy is also associated with higher goal challenges, decisions involving choice, greater effort and commitment to goals, persistence, and resilience. Although strong self-efficacy beliefs are highly resistant and predictable (Pajares, 2002), the character and extent of perceived self-efficacy can change, becoming stronger throughout life. Perceived self-efficacy is influenced by environmental factors, such as new information, expectations, and the support of others (Van der Bijl & Shortridge-Baggett, 2001). It is important to note that, self-efficacy beliefs are more easily weakened through negative appraisals than they are strengthened through positive encouragement (Pajares, 2002).

Sources of information that can influence self-efficacy include:

1. *Successful mastery*—resulting from practice; or interpreting the results of previous performances or experiences. "Persons who are certain of their capacities tend to attribute failure to situational factors like not enough effort or bad strategy" (Van der Bijl & Shortridge-Baggett, 2001, p. 192).
2. *Vicarious experiences*—including observing the performance of others or modeling.
3. *Social persuasion*—convincing individuals through praise and encouragement. "By giving instructions, suggestions, and advice, health care professionals try to con-

vince persons that they can succeed in a difficult task" (Van der Bijl & Shortridge-Baggett, 2001, p. 192).

4. *Somatic and emotional states*—positive mood heightens self-efficacy, reducing stress reactions and tempering negative emotional responses.

Self-efficacy has proven to be a more consistent predictor of behavioral outcomes than any other motivational construct (Pajares, 2002). Outcomes of self-efficacy include indices of physical (e.g., vitality), psychological (e.g., feelings of accomplishment), and social (e.g., group participation) well-being (Berarducci & Lengacher, 1998). To increase client well-being, the nurse should focus on improving emotional, cognitive, or motivational processes, increasing behavioral competencies, or altering the social conditions under which clients live and work.

Agency

The concept of agency has many similarities with capability and can be defined as "the freedom of individual human beings to make choices and to act on these choices in ways that make a difference in their lives" (Martin, Sugarman, and Thompson, 2003, p. 1). "Self-agency is defined as the conceptual understanding of self as an agent capable of shaping motives, behavior, and future possibilities" (DeSocio, Kitzman, and Cole, 2003, p. 20).

Agency requires internal intent, belief, and desire, and external actions to overcome constraints and threats to autonomy. Additionally, personal efficacy beliefs mediate agency through the interaction resulting from capacity (component of power) and trying (intention-directed effort) (Morris, Menon, and Ames, 2001). Agency involves deliberate actions to achieve goals including setting goals, planning a course of action, and persisting despite distractions and obstacles. Nurses can use empathetic relationships to inspire hope that change is possible, and offer a context for self-understanding. Self-understanding is necessary for clients to envision and commit to purposeful behavior and a desired future self.

Agency is based on deliberate reflection, choice, and freedom of action, and is influenced by self-determination and efficacy. Freedom of choice provides multiple alternatives for action. Freedom of action means "being able to do that which one chooses to do" (Martin et al., 2003, p. 47). Self-determination is the exercising of voluntary control over personal actions.

Environment is an important influence on agency. Environments that prompt and mobilize self-agency are those supplying adequate resources, supportive relationships, and opportunities to exercise self-influence. In contrast, environments that suppress aspirations and threaten basic needs hinder self-development by causing disruptive emotional states and limiting opportunities (DeSocio et al., 2003). Other factors that might determine individual choices and actions include explicit coercion, physical-biological states and processes, sociocultural rules and practices, unconscious processes over which the individual has no control, and random events.

Agency is based on purposeful action. Western cultures believe in an independent-self where agency is experienced by expressing internal needs, rights, and capacities in order to withstand undue social pressure. In Western cultures, "personal agency assumes that people will both perceive themselves as the origins of their own behavior and be motivated to act upon opportunities that allow one to be the sole initiator of their behavior" (Hernandez & Iyenger, 2001, p. 270). By contrast, Eastern cultures see thought and behavior as being interdependent, and originating from the collective culture. In these cultures, agency is experienced as being receptive of others, adjusting to their needs and demands, and restraining personal inner needs or desires (Hernandez & Iyenger, 2001). Different cultural views of the individual inherently imply different assignments of control, authority, and stability. In Western cultures these actions are attributed to the individual, whereas Eastern cultures attribute them to the greater social collective. Westerners seek choice, control, and self-determination. Personal aspirations are conditioned by the norms of the individual's most familiar social groups. When the social context is associated with poverty and social disadvantage, life experiences may stifle personal aspirations and negate beliefs in an individual's ability to purposefully change future outcomes through self-effort (DeSocio et al., 2003).

Nursing interventions to increase perceived agency should support behavior change and can consist of structured activities, such as envisioning possibilities, developing goals, devising plans, preparing through cognitive review, practicing behavior within the appropriate context, and evaluating the effectiveness of behavior (DeSocio et al., 2003). Nurses should help clients see themselves as the source of change, apart from the collaborative relationship provided by the nurse. Doing so prepares the client to act with conviction and to take responsibility for self-regulated change.

Self-Care Agency

Self-care agency has been defined as the actions taken by the individual for self-care, a concept popularized by Orem (1995). Individuals are assumed to have the cognitive, psychomotor, and emotional skills needed to engage in operations that are essential to self-care and ensure maintenance of health and well-being (Carter, 1998). Self-care agency is defined as "the power to engage in the estimative and productive operations of self-care" (Gast el al., 1989). Self-care agency thus emphasizes the capability to carry out actions. Dimensions of self-care agency, as described by Kearney & Fleischer (1979), include an active response to situations; motivation; a knowledge base; and a feeling of self-worth.

Personal traits provide the ability to perform self-care actions. According to the Nursing Development Conference Group (1979), personal traits can be divided among basic personal abilities, enabling traits, and operational traits. Basic personal abilities include sensation, perception, memory, and orientation, and are related to the client's ability to perform any type of deliberate action. Enabling traits (or power components) are related to the client's ability to engage in self-care. And operational traits (or self-care operations) include the client's ability to observe conditions and factors in the immediate environment that are significant to self-care (estimative operations); make judgments and decisions about what can, should, and will be done to provide self-care (productive operations); and take actions to meet self-care needs (productive operations).

Easom (2003) suggests that perceived self-efficacy and barriers affect the self-care abilities of older adults, especially the ability to take responsibility and initiative in promoting their own health and functioning.

Competence

Capability has no action component and is defined as the global belief that individuals have about their ability to achieve desired goals. In contrast, self-efficacy and competence are action-oriented concepts. Self-efficacy refers to an individual's perceived ability (capacity) to perform a specific behavior, and competence is a judgment of demonstrated adequate or proficient skill, ability, or performance in a specific domain (e.g., language, social situations, work environments). Competence is an achieved capacity resulting from action-oriented behaviors.

Weinert (2001, p. 56) argues that "competence and competencies should be understood primarily as the mental conditions necessary for cognitive, social, and vocational achievement." Consequently, competence is restricted to domain-specific learning, content-specific, task-specific, and/or demand-specific performance dispositions, and specific functional competencies, such as memory, problem-solving, and learning or skills, knowledge, and strategies.

Competence can be demonstrated through concepts, procedures, or by performing tasks. Conceptual competence is related to rule-based, abstract knowledge about an entire domain. Procedural competence relates to procedures and skills applied in concrete situations. Performance competence involves skills needed to evaluate situations and devise solutions including general problem-solving abilities; critical thinking skills; domain-general and domain-specific knowledge; realistic, positive self-confidence, and social competencies (Weinert, 2001).

Consequently, specific knowledge and skills are needed for competence. Personal control beliefs, achievement motive, and self-concept contribute to motivation for competence. The relationship between competence and performance is moderated by cognitive style, memory capacity, and familiarity with the task situation among other variables.

MULTICULTURAL COMPETENCE

According to Marcus and Kitayama (1994) (see Chapter 1), each individual is embedded within a variety of sociocultural contexts or cultures, such as country or region of origin, ethnicity, religion, gender, family, birth cohort, or profession. Each of these cultural contexts makes some claim on the individual and is associated with a set of ideas and practices about how to behave.

Westerners perceive themselves as being able to stand apart and be separate from others in their environment. They find it more natural to describe themselves in terms of the singular 'I', an entity that is context-free, because they perceive themselves as possessing traits that are distinctive and independent of their social roles. Individuals are expected to express independence from others, identify and express their unique attributes, and remain relatively unaffected by group and environmental pressures (Hernandez & Iyengar, 2001).

By contrast, individuals from Eastern cultures see themselves as interconnected with and interrelated to others in their social context. The focal point is not the inner self, but rather the relationships the individual has with others. Experiencing interdependence means individuals see themselves as part of an encompassing social relationship. In this context individuals recognize that their behavior is largely determined by the thoughts, feelings, and actions of others in the social relationship. Interdependent-selves do not strive for independence but instead pursue the goal of fitting in and conforming to the demands and expectations of their social groups (Hernandez & Iyengar, 2001).

As a consequence, while American culture primarily conceptualizes agency as a property of individuals, other cultures (e.g., Chinese) conceptualize agency primarily in terms of collectives such as family or organizational groups or nonhuman deities or fate (Morris et al., 2001). "In Chinese culture, hierarchical role relationships, for example the exchange of paternal benevolence for filial piety, restrict individual agency and structure many interactions, even those in modern work organizations (Morris et al., 2001). In Chinese culture family influence dominates. But in Japanese culture corporate agency is often more prominent than family influence. These examples of cultural differences reiterate the need for a basic understanding of the many influences affecting the needs and choices of clients.

References

Bandura, A. (1986). *Social foundations of thought and action. A social cognitive theory.* Englewood Cliffs, NJ: Prentice-Hall.

Bandura, A. (1994). Self-efficacy. In V. H. Ramachandran (Ed.), *Encyclopedia of human behavior* (vol. 4, pp. 71–81). San Diego, CA: Academic Press.

Bandura, A. (1997). *Self-efficacy: The exercise of control.* New York: Freeman.

Berarducci, A., & Lengacher, C. A. (1998). Self-efficacy: An essential component of advanced-practice nursing. *Nursing Connections, 11,* 55–67.

Carter, P. A. (1998). Self-care agency: The concept and how it is measured. *Journal of Nursing Measurement, 6,* 195–207.

DeSocio, J., Kitzman, H., & Cole, R. (2003). Testing the relationship between self-agency and enactment of health behaviors. *Research in Nursing and Health, 26,* 20–29.

Easom, L. R. (2003). Perceived self-efficacy and barriers in older adults. *Journal of Gerontological Nursing, 29,* 11–19.

Gast, H., Denyes, M., Campbell, J., Hartwag, D., Schott-Baer, D., & Isenberg, M. (1989). Self-care agency: Conceptualizations and operationalizations. *Advances in Nursing Science, 12,* 26–38.

Herdandez, M., & Iyenger, S. S. (2001). What drives whom? A cultural perspective on human agency. *Social Cognition, 19,* 269–294.

Kearney, B., & Fleischer, B. (1979). Development of an instrument to measure exercise of self-care agency. *Research in Nursing and Health, 2,* 25–34.

Marcus, H. R., & Kitayama, S. (1994). The cultural shaping of emotion: A conceptual framework. In. S. Kitayama & H. R. Marcus (Eds.), *Emotion and culture: Empirical studies of mutual influence* (pp. 339–351). Washington DC: American Psychological Association.

Martin, J., Sugarman, J., & Thompson, J. (2003). *Psychology and the question of agency.* New York: SUNY.

Morris, M. W., Menon, T., & Ames, D. R. (2001). Culturally conferred conceptions of agency: A key to social perception of persons, groups, and other actors. *Personality and Social Psychology Review, 5,* 169–182.

Orem, D. E. (1995). *Nursing: Concepts of practice* (5th ed.). St. Louis: Mosby.

Pajares, F. (2002). Overview of social cognitive theory and of self-efficacy. Retrieved 5/10/04 from http://www.emory.edu/EDUCATION/mfp/eff.html.

Ryan, R. M., & Deci, E. L. (2000). Self-determination theory and the facilitation of intrinsic motivation, social development, and well-being. *American Psychologist, 55,* 68–78.

Soukhanov, A. (Ed.). (1992). *The American Heritage Dictionary.* Boston: Houghton Mifflin.

Van der Bijl, J. J., & Shortridge-Baggett, L. M. (2001). The theory and measurement of the self-efficacy construct. *Scholarly Inquiry for Nursing Practice: An International Journal, 15,* 189–205.

Weinert, F. E. (2001). Concept of competence: A conceptual clarification. In D. S. Rychen & L. H. Salganik (Eds.), *Defining and selecting key competencies* (pp. 45–65). Seattle, WA: Wogrefe & Huber.

CHAPTER 7

Power Part Two: Control

Concepts
Manageability
Self-Regulation

Models and Theories
Neuman's Health-Care Systems Model
Locus of Control
Stress and Coping

Helpful Lists
Assessment of Perceived Control,
    pg. 91

Descriptors of Control, pgs. 92–93
Components of Control, pg. 93
Types of Coping, pg. 96
Cognitive Activities that Aid in Coping,
    pg. 97
Positive Outcomes of Coping,
    pg. 98
Strategies to Promote Self-Regulation,
    pg. 99
Interventions to Enhance Perception
    of Control, pg. 101

Thought Questions

1. Does perceived control differ from actual control? If so, how? Can you give some examples?
2. What are the differences between personal control and external control? Why is this distinction important?
3. Is coping a strength? Why or why not?
4. Identify several cultural differences in perceived control and describe their effect on nursing interventions.
5. How can intrinsic motivation and control be enhanced in nursing practice?

Chapter Synopsis

This chapter introduces the concept of control as a human strength and as an aspect of power in the Healthiness Theory. Control is closely related to other concepts in the Healthiness Theory, such as goals, connection, choice, challenge, and capacity. Neuman's health-care systems model, locus of control, and stress and coping theories are described, as are the concepts related to control, such as manageability and self-regulation. The importance of multicultural competency is again stressed. Finally, some broad intervention strategies are presented.

CONTROL

Personal control consists of an individual's beliefs and expectations about how to effectively shape and alter the environment to bring about positive events and avoid negative ones (Peterson & Stunkard, 1989; Ross & Sastry, 1999). In the Healthiness Theory (see Chapter 2), control is closely related to choice, confidence, and capability, all concepts that are part of power in the theory.

Perceived control is "the expectation of having the power to participate in making decisions in order to obtain desirable consequences and a sense of personal competence in a given situation" (Rodin, 1990, p. 4). Consequently, individuals feel that they are influential (rather than helpless) in making decisions and affecting outcomes. By exercising imagination, knowledge, skill, and choice they see themselves affecting a structured and responsive environment.

Perceived control has been understood as a composite of contingency beliefs (outcome expectancy), competence beliefs (expectation of efficacy), and control expectancy (the domains in which perceived control operates) (Grob, 2000). "The expectancy component refers to generalized cognitive estimates of the amount of control one possesses, whereas the appraisal component refers to the valuation or perceived importance of the situation at stake" (Grob, 2000, p. 333). In other words, individuals think about how much personal control they have when evaluating circumstances.

Skinner (1996) suggests that components of control include agent-ends relations, such as perceived control, personal control, and sense of control; agent-means relations, such as capability, beliefs about agency and capacity, and self-efficacy; and means-ends relations, such as locus of control, attributions, and responsibility.

Personal control is a learned and generalized expectation that events and circumstances result from personal choices and actions. Individuals with high levels of control use persistence and attention to address problems, and are more likely to act when difficulties arise. In contrast, low levels of control undermine the individual's will and motivation to cope actively with problems (Sastry & Ross, 1998). Intellectual, emotional, behavioral, and physiological vigor in the face of challenging situations and events is associated with high personal control (Peterson & Stunkard, 1989).

Personal control is a cognitive appraisal of "the perceived ability to significantly alter events" (Skinner, 1996, p. 549), and includes expectations about making decisions in a given situation in order to obtain desirable consequences and a sense of personal competence (Rodin, 1990). But perception of personal control may not match the objective data. Objective or actual control uses selective responses to regulate or influence the attainment, maintenance, or the avoidance of intended outcomes (Grob, 2000; Rodin, 1990). Objective control involves the ability to regulate or influence intended outcomes (Rodin, 1990). The degree of personal control may be affected by chance, luck, fate, powerful others, or beliefs associated with an external locus of control (discussed later in this chapter). Ideally, what individuals think they can control (perceived control) will match what they can control (actual control).

Belief about control can be a cognitive appraisal in a specific context (situational), or a general, global, dispositional belief (Lazarus & Folkman, 1984). Situational control appraisals are domain specific and are based on the value of various domains (e.g., health, work) to the individual. It is similar to self-efficacy, and involves the belief that individuals can shape and influence a particular human-environment process. Situational control is socially structured and transmitted, and views the individual as multidimensional and open to learning and change. Control can also be classified as global, which involves "a belief that in general individuals are able to control the conditions of their lives" (Pearlin & Pioli, 2003). Global control is related to long-term outcomes rather than the short-term control exerted in domain-specific situations.

Perceived control is the judgment that individuals can obtain desired outcomes and avoid undesirable ones (Thompson, 2002). A potentially negative event is not as stressful when it is accompanied by a belief in personal control. For example, an individual diagnosed with a life-altering disease may feel less overwhelmed if they feel that something they can do (e.g., reduce stress, alter their diet) can reduce symptoms, improve quality of life, and even affect their prognosis. Perceived control is associated with positive emotions, leads to active problem-solving, reduces anxiety in the form of stress, and buffers against negative psychological responses (Thompson, 2002). Perceived control consists of two parts: locus (internal or external) of control, and self-efficacy (Thompson, 2002). Making progress toward goals is an important source of perceived control and general well-being.

Control does not have to be realistic to be beneficial. The illusion of control, even over objectively random events, has a positive effect on various types of behavior. Self-fulfilling prophecies diminish threats and reduce barriers resulting in greater perceived control, reduced stress, increased motivation, and enhanced performance (Peterson & Stunkard, 1989). Actions effective in overcoming threats to perceived control include alliances with groups and collectives, social support, higher power appeals, and negotiation.

A balanced sense of control helps adaptive planning, since individuals with too high a sense of control may not plan due to a false sense of security, and individuals with too low a sense of control may not plan because they assume they cannot influence the outcome (Clark-Plaskie & Lachman, 1999).

Perceived control can affect the belief that individuals can cause or influence the occurrence, timing, or extent of actual outcomes; choose among outcomes; cope with the consequences of outcomes and/or understand these outcomes (Peterson, 1999). In order to assess a client's level of perceived control, it is important to understand that perceived control:

1. Results from the client's relationship with the world. It is not simply an individual disposition, and it is not simply an objective property of an environment.
2. Is measured by self-report. Nurses can ask direct questions about perceived control, because it is determined by how the client feels about their level of control.
3. Is desirable (when the environment is favorable) because it encourages emotional, motivational, behavioral, and physiological vigor in the face of demands (Peterson, 1999).
4. Is stimulated by novel and challenging events and is particularly important in the face of overwhelming negative events.
5. Is impeded by failure and encouraged by success, although it does not bear a one-to-one relationship to past patterns of success and failure (Peterson, 1999). Perceived control and persistence are not effective in unresponsive settings.
6. Is difficult to use when choices are too numerous, too complex, or too difficult (Peterson, 1999).

Choice, agency, and feelings of self-determination are central elements supporting the intrinsic motivation to achieve (Rodin, 1990). Appraised high control leads to information seeking, planning, strategizing, preventative efforts, and direct action, because all of these actions can be effective in exerting personal control (Skinner, 1996).

Losses of subjective or objective control can result in both primary and secondary control. Primary control means influencing the environment in order to produce the desired outcomes (Weise, 1990). Primary control is behavior control and may be associated with strategies ranging from tenacious goal pursuit to helplessness in which circumstances are changed in accordance with personal preferences (Clark-Plaskie & Lachman, 1999). In indirect primary control, conditions are modified not through direct confrontation, but through methods to modify the behavior of others (Skaff & Gardiner, 2003). For example, in 2005, the parents of Terry Schiavo, a woman in a permanently vegetative state, sought to supersede state and federal court decisions to have her feeding tube removed by lobbying the United States Congress to mandate that her feeding tube be reinserted.

Secondary control (or coping) is an effort to control the psychological impact of the objective conditions (Weise, 1990) by using strategies ranging from flexible goal adjustment to rigid perseverance and relinquishments, to adjusting personal preferences to the situation. Secondary control is cognitive control where "The intent is to control the self's reactions to the conditions or situations confronted, to alter the self, and fit in with the environment rather than try to change the environment" (Skaff & Gardiner, 2003). In secondary coping, individuals feel less like helpless victims because they have accepted the circumstances. Secondary control is often associated with emotion-focused coping. Antecedents of control include information, choice, and predictability. For example, decision control involves choice, the belief that the individual alone selects both the desired goals and the strategies to obtain them (Rodin, 1990).

Control may vary on different dimensions, including *agents* of control (individual or group); *means* or mechanisms (behavioral or cognitive action, accessing others, and objective realities of the environment, such as opportunities and barriers); and *ends* or targets that may be inner attributes (desires, personal goals, emotions), or environmental (occurrence of events, reactions to the repercussions of events) (Skaff & Gardiner, 2003).

A number of control descriptors have been identified including:

- *Indirect control*—appealing to more effective forces for intercession (e.g., through parents or school officials to decrease drug use among adolescents).
- *Purposive supplication*—using "higher power" chains of control (e.g., prayer).
- *Self-control*—controlling emotions and impulses and how individuals present themselves (Pearlin & Pioli, 2003).
- *Sociopolitical context*—includes objective differences in power and control.
- *Collective control*—where members are largely anonymous, engage in few interpersonal exchanges, and outcome expectations are beyond the reach of individual attainment (e.g., lobbying a legislator). Collective action occurs through participation and identification with the group (Pearlin & Pioli, 2003).
- *Predictive control*—predicting adverse events in order to avoid disappointment. This may involve *illusory* control, where individuals align with the forces of chance in uncontrollable or chance-determined situations (e.g., predicting survival in a life-threatening situation); *vicarious* control, achieved by associating with power-

ful others; or *interpretive* control where events are interpreted for better understanding.

- *Role-specific mastery*—is closely related to agency, the individual's ability to act on their own behalf, and to yield or share control when negotiating with others (e.g., negotiations that may occur in the client-nurse relationship).
- *Function-specific mastery*—"the patterns of activity that are associated with the sat-isfaction of daily needs and natural tendencies" (e.g., taking of medications as pre-scribed) (Pearlin & Pioli, 2003, p. 14).

Control can also be described in terms of contingency (likelihood), competence (capacity), and expectancy (confidence) to cause an intended event (Weise, 1990). Each of these components is related to control in the following ways:

- Low contingency and low competence is associated with secondary or relinquished control (e.g., doing what an authority such as the nurse or physician says, even though the client may not want to).
- High contingency and low competence is associated with primary or secondary control in which the individual tries to increase competence (e.g., seeking informa-tion in order to decide whether or not to accept the nurse's suggested interven-tion).
- Low contingency and high competence is associated with secondary control, or primary control if contingency can be changed (e.g., influencing a family member to "tell" the nurse that the client does not want to accept the intervention).
- Only high contingency and high competence is associated with primary control (e.g., the client decides to use a different strategy).

It has been shown that intrinsic motivation can be increased through the lack of important external constraints and the presence of choice. Rodin (1990) also found that choice and feelings of self-determination are important to intrinsic motivation. Intellectual, emotional, behavioral, and physiological vigor in the face of challenging situations and events is associated with high personal control (Peterson & Stunkard, 1989).

Increasing intrinsic motivation enhances the perception of competence by involving individuals in tasks that create interest, challenge, and novelty (Ryan, 1982). Effects of control may be *cognitive,* self-directing plans and goals; *motivational,* enhancing perse-verance and endurance; *emotional,* cognitively mediating anxiety; and *choice enhancing* by evaluating environments the individual is capable of handling (Rodin, 1990).

Control can be driven by demands rather than by choices and personal goals (Deci & Ryan, 1985). Demands lead to pressure and tension, and result in either compli-ance with or defiance toward the source of the demands. Consequently, control impera-tives include: should, have to, ought to, and must, all resulting in conflict and power struggle. Motivation initiated and regulated by forces wholly beyond the individual's control leads to a sense of personal helplessness. This results in the individual being unable to achieve the desired results. This information is useful to the nurse-client rela-tionship because the nurse can thwart potential power struggles by avoiding control imperatives.

A number of correlates have been associated with control. High levels of control are associated with high socioeconomic status (SES), high levels of income and education, being employed in complex, nonroutine, autonomous (self-directed), and well compensated jobs (Sastry & Ross, 1998). Low socioeconomic status is related to relatively greater external control beliefs (less personal control), whereas higher levels of income enhance resources and options, promoting internal control beliefs (greater personal control).

Controllability is associated with predictability, which is defined as a sense of coherence or permanence. Experiencing a lack of control and powerlessness can have a lasting impact on beliefs about what can and cannot be controlled, attitudes about who is in control, and what kinds of control are possible given the circumstances and the context (Skaff & Gardiner, 2003). Being in control, a condition where things are under the individual's control, requires both environmental support and individual initiatives (Syme, 1990).

All external events can be viewed as having two functional aspects: an informational or feedback aspect, and a controlling aspect (Ryan, 1982). An environmental event that is informational provides behaviorally relevant information without pressure for a particular outcome. Further, verbal encouragement that does not imply pressure to attain particular outcomes but does encourage successful outcomes may enhance client interest in the activity (Ryan, 1982). However, the fit between the individual and the environment is critical. Clients must believe in their personal competence and effectiveness, but must also be aware of their limitations and the influence of outside factors (Clark-Plaskie & Lachman, 1999).

Differences in explaining bad events are determined by the individual's explanatory style (Peterson, 1999). A flexible, accommodating explanatory style can buffer the negative effects of age-typical problems (Clark-Plaskie & Lachman, 1999). Both the young-old and the old-old have been found to have a moderate sense of mastery, with education positively related to mastery in both groups, sense of coherence (SOC) (comprehensibility, manageability, and meaningfulness), and mastery related to health status in both groups, SOC and self-esteem correlated with perceived health in the young-old, and mastery correlated with perceived health in the old-old (Forbes, 2001). Older adults have a lower sense of internal beliefs (personal control) and higher external beliefs (external control) in general, and for health and intellectual functioning, than young and middle-aged adults, and perceived control decreases with age at an accelerating rate (Clark-Plaskie & Lachman, 1999; Ross & Sastry, 1999). This information can help nurses understand why many older patients experience feelings of little personal control, and therefore seem unable to change their circumstances.

The relationship between work experiences and perceived control in midlife seems to be a reciprocal one. Middle-aged adults perceive higher internal control for goals in the work domain than for goals in the family, health, leisure, and financial domains. Women have higher levels of external control beliefs. It has been suggested that women may have a lower sense of control over their lives than men when influenced by economic dependency, restricted opportunities, role overload, and the routine nature of housework and women's jobs (Ross & Sastry, 1999). Students who have high control beliefs prefer programs in which they can set their own goals and control their own pace, whereas those low in control prefer programs with goals already assigned and a pace already imposed (Peterson & Stunkard, 1989).

THEORIES

Neuman's Health-Care Systems Model

In Neuman's Health-Care Systems Model, consistent with the stability view of health, the purpose of nursing is to "assist clients to retain, attain, or maintain system stability" (Neuman, 2002, p. 25). Neuman's model emphasizes control of intrapersonal, interpersonal, and extrapersonal stressors. Resistance to stressors is provided by a flexible line of defense, a dynamic protective buffer made up of all variables affecting the individual at any given moment. These variables may include the individual's physiological structure and condition, sociocultural background, spiritual beliefs, developmental state, cognitive skills, age, and gender. If the flexible line of defense is unable to protect the individual, the stressor breaks through, disturbing the individual's equilibrium, and triggering a reaction. The reaction may lead toward restoration of balance or toward death, depending on the lines of resistance that attempt to restore balance. The reaction to the stressor and the prognosis are affected by:

- The number and strength of the stressors affecting the individual.
- The length of time individual is affected.
- The meaningfulness of the stressor for the individual.

This model is consistent with primary, secondary, and tertiary prevention nursing activities to reduce stress factors and strengthen the client's resistance (e.g., control stressors or the individual's response).

Locus of Control

Rotter (1966), as part of his Social Learning Theory, proposed that control beliefs can be differentiated on the basis of perceived locus of control (perceived source of control as internal or external). According to Rotter, individuals with an external locus of control consider outcomes to be unpredictable because of luck, chance, or fate, or from being under the control of powerful others. Individuals who are defensive externals (defensive with an external locus of control) become very active in competitive situations because they fear failure, whereas passive externals (passive with an external locus of control) become more passive toward events. In contrast, individuals with an internal locus of control view outcomes as contingent on their own behavior or as relatively permanent characteristics. Individuals who are bilocal believe that both internal and external forces exercise control. Consequently, individuals who are bilocal change what they can and accept what cannot be changed (Fournier & Jeanrie, 2003). Nurses should observe and interview clients and their families when assessing which style of control best represents a client. This information will help the nurse understand the way a client responds to circumstances. Knowing that a client is a defensive external can explain a sense of competition, and observing that client is passive external can explain a lack of response.

In contrast, Fournier & Jeanrie (2003) proposed a five-part division of locus of control beliefs: *defeatist* (outcomes are determined by context and others); *dependent* (outcomes are determined by chance and fate); *prescriptive* (outcomes are determined by social norms and dictates); *responsible* (outcomes are determined by personal actions);

and *proactive* (outcomes are determined by personal efforts and environmental contingencies).

Locus of control is primarily situation-specific, reflecting beliefs of capability in particular situations. In this regard, locus of control resembles self-efficacy. "Self-efficacy focuses upon the individual's belief that he or she can effectively perform a specific action whereas control focuses on the belief that certain actions will achieve ultimately desired goals" (Ross & Sastry, 1999, p. 372). Behavior to satisfy a valued need depends more on the individual's attitude toward the situation than on the situation itself. This attitude is shaped by perceptions of an individual's capacities to influence outcomes (Fournier & Jeanrie, 2003, p. 140).

Stress and Coping (Loss and Threat)

It is unclear whether autonomy, self-determination, and perceived freedom are within or outside the domain of control (Skinner, 1996). Because autonomy is described as self-direction undertaken without outside control, it is not discussed in this chapter. "Self-determination refers to the experience of freedom in initiating one's behavior" (Skinner, 1996, p. 557), and is therefore discussed in Chapter 8. Self-efficacy and agency beliefs have some similarities with control beliefs and are discussed in Chapter 6.

Coping is a response to stress. A primary function of coping has been described as the "regulation of distress and the management of problems causing the distress" (Folkman & Moskowitz, 2000, p. 647). The stress and coping literature has dealt almost exclusively with negative (e.g., threat) events and their outcomes. But recently there has been consideration of proactive coping, the ability to see that stressful situations, when viewed as challenges, might have a favorable outcome (see Chapter 9). Can coping then be considered a positive resource for health? Reframing and infusing ordinary events with positive meaning (proactive coping strategies) are associated with positive outcomes, such as stress-related growth, positive personal changes, and meaning-making (Somerfield & McCrae, 2003). However, the essence of coping is still a *reaction* to a negatively appraised event or situation.

Folkman & Moskowitz, 2000; Fredrickson, 2001; Lazarus and Folkman, 1984; and Schwarzer and Knoll, 2003, identify many types of coping, including:

- *Instrumental coping* involves reframing a situation in a positive light and is attentive, vigilant, and/or confrontational; compared to *emotional coping,* which tends be avoidant and/or palliative.
- *Problem-focused coping* involves mastery by directing efforts toward solving or managing a problem by using instrumental, situation-specific, and task-oriented actions compared with *emotion-focused coping,* which includes thought or actions to relieve the emotional impact of stress.
- *Assimilative coping* involves modifying the environment whereas *accommodative coping* involves self modification.
- *Reactive coping* involves a response to harm or loss experienced in the past (e.g., an accident) in comparison to *anticipatory coping,* which deals with an imminent threat in the near future (e.g., retirement or an exam).
- *Preventive coping* foreshadows an uncertain threat potential in the distant future (e.g., job loss or illness), whereas *proactive coping* deals with challenges that are

potentially self-promoting (e.g., goal management instead of risk management), where demanding situations are viewed as personal challenges, and ordinary events are infused with positive meaning.

Relational meaning refers to the significance of an emotional encounter and is the immediate cause of experienced or displayed emotions. Individuals construct meaning by appraising or evaluating the personal significance of what happens during an encounter. Each emotion has a distinctively different relational meaning (Lazarus, 2003b). In emotion-focused coping, no attempt is made to change the situation and the individual may reappraise the problem more benignly than it actually is. In contrast, problem-focused coping involves a positive reappraisal of the circumstances, which includes focusing on the good in what has happened or is happening; managing thoughts and behaviors to solve the underlying cause of the distress; and creating positive events by giving ordinary events a positive meaning (Larsen, Hemenover, Norris, and Cacioppo, 2003). "Being able to put a positive spin on a harsh fate can motivate problem-solving efforts, self-actualization, and the enjoyment of life in spite of negative realities" (Lazarus, 2003a, p. 105).

If the individual's beliefs and goals do not match the meaning of a situation, they will experience distress, and will try to either cope or eradicate the source of the distress. Individuals often try to reduce the incongruence between the appraised meaning of a situation and their preexisting beliefs and goals (global meaning). Reattributions, changing global beliefs and generating new valued goals, are all ways to adjust meaning (Park & Folkman, 1998). Several cognitive activities can be used to describe the emotions that aid in coping with stress:

1. Vigilant strategies neutralize distress by refocusing attention (e.g., jogging, taking a holiday).
2. Escape avoidance strategies use wishful thinking and tension reduction (e.g., eating, drinking, and sleeping too much).
3. Altering the subjective meaning of the circumstance, through humor or denial, releases tension and prevents the catastrophizing of events. But this can result in the client denying the severity of a problem and avoiding appropriate action. When this happens it is helpful for the nurse to remain on task, reaffirm the issues, and encourage clients to get more information so they can deal with reality.

In addition to reappraising events, individuals can change the meaning of a situation through a number of other cognitive coping strategies. These coping strategies include compensatory self-enhancement (focusing on or exaggerating another individual's capacities or virtues or those of an unrelated domain), downward comparisons (judging themselves as well off compared with others), and developing a different perspective on the situation. Other strategies include taking a long-term perspective, maintaining a sense of humor, and remembering or focusing on events that reinforce existing beliefs and goals (Park & Folkman, 1998).

Threats to an individual's self-concept are often reduced when the event is seen as a "wake-up call" indicating that priorities and goals need to be reevaluated. This often results in individuals reordering priorities and revising life goals as they reappraise the event as an opportunity for growth (challenge) rather than as a loss (Davis, Nolen-Hoeksema, and Larson, 1998). Perceiving that something positive resulted from an experience ("a wake-up call") appears to influence adjustment more than changes in the ability to make sense of a loss (Davis et al., 1998).

Making sense of or *finding meaning in* may refer to the extent individuals have reconciled their appraised (or reappraised) meaning of an event with their beliefs about global meaning (Park & Folkman, 1998). Positive outcomes of confronting stressful experiences and coping effectively include:

1. *Enhanced social resources*—including developing a confidential relationship, better relationships with family members and friends, and forming new support networks.
2. *Enhanced personal resources*—including cognitive and intellectual differentiation, self-reliance and self-understanding; empathy, altruism, and maturity; and changes in basic values and priorities.
3. *Development of new coping skills*—including cognitive coping skills, problem-solving and help-seeking skills, and being able to regulate and control affect.

RELATED CONCEPTS

Manageability

Manageability (part of SOC, see following) is defined as "the extent to which individuals perceive that they have the personal and social resources to confront and cope with demand" (Korotkov, 1998, p. 55). This definition indicates that manageability may be before or a consequence of perceived control.

The sense of coherence (SOC) comprises three intertwined constructs, manageability, comprehensibility, and meaningfulness (Antonovsky, 1987). Antonovsky proposed that the SOC is shaped by the extent that generalized resources (e.g., social support, strengths such as goals and connectedness) provide meaningful, orderly, and coherent life experiences. The SOC is defined as a dispositional orientation as well as a generalized way of viewing the world, and is "a global orientation that is reasonably stable by the end of early adulthood" (Korotkov, 1998, p. 55). A strong SOC helps individuals to actively cope with negative stressors.

Self-Regulation

Self-regulation can be defined as a goal-related sequence of actions and/or steering processes (Moes & Gebhardt, 2000). According to Zimmerman (2000), self-regulation is associated with planned and cyclically adapted, goal-related, self-generated thought, feelings, and actions. Self-regulation is an interaction of behavioral, environmental, and personal processes. *Behavioral* self-regulation involves self observation and the strategic adjustment of performance processes, such as an individual's method of learning. *Environmental* self-regulation refers to observing and adjusting environmental conditions or outcomes. Covert *personal* self-regulation entails monitoring and adjusting cognitive and affective states, such as using imagery for remembering or relaxing.

It has been suggested that humans possess two inherent, overarching goals: survival and coherence. Goals vary in terms of importance and individuals tend to be more committed to highly important goals. Goals also vary in difficulty of accomplishment. For optimum achievement, it is helpful if a goal is not too difficult or too easy. Goals also vary on a temporal level, whether they are reachable within a specified time frame. An individual must be conscious of the specific goal in order to be motivated toward its accomplishment and must believe that the environment or context will support goal achievement.

The motivation to change occurs when individuals want to reduce discrepancies between their perceived state and a desired state (Moes & Gebhardt, 2000). An example would be a smoker with the risk of developing lung cancer (perceived state), giving up smoking and becoming a nonsmoker with a decreased risk (desired state). Goal orientation requires individuals to be self-focused and action oriented. However, different goals may require different strategies, such as approach or avoidance strategies, action or reactive orientation, and maintenance or change approaches. Regulation of goals may be achievement-directed (e.g., losing weight to stay healthy) or emotion-oriented (e.g., eating to feel good). Emotions help to regulate and energize behavior, including continuing behavior with positive outcomes and inhibiting behavior with negative outcomes. Emotional responses are crucial motivational elements that affect direct responses to appraisals of goal-related progress, experiences to be regulated, and influences on cognitions and behaviors (Cameron & Leventhal, 2003).

Cognitive strategies to promote self-regulation are based on the assumption that although emotions aren't controllable, the thoughts that underlie them are (Weise, 1990). Consequently, cognitive strategies that nurses can use to promote client self-regulation include:

1. *Alteration of time frame*—redirecting thoughts from bleak present to bright future
2. *Selective attribution*—attributing cause to external rather than internal factors
3. *Selective ignoring*—looking at good things
4. *Positive comparisons*—thinking of others who are worse off
5. *Selective valuation*—deciding that "x" was not important

MULTICULTURAL COMPETENCY

The single most important determinant of personal control may be the cultural norms concerning collective control (Peterson & Stunkard, 1989). Groups of individuals may possess a sense of control based on a shared purpose. Prediction of shared control is greatly enhanced by simultaneously taking into account both personal and situational characteristics (Peterson & Stunkard, 1989).

African Americans have comparatively low levels of personal control (possibly associated with socioeconomic factors) but similar (to other Americans) levels of self-esteem (possibly related to strong interpersonal relationships). However, it is difficult to disentangle the effects of socioeconomic status on sense of control from those of race and ethnicity (Skaff & Gardiner, 2003). Secondary control strategies are used more frequently in Eastern cultures, and primary personal control is at the core of the American value system.

Individuals who are high in personal agency are more action-oriented in coping with problems, more likely to limit negative psychological reactions when confronted with stressful conditions, more capable of rallying other resources to resist stress, and are more likely to meet their goals. Those high in communal mastery are more likely to approach challenges or problems by relating to others, rather than alone or by competing with others. This translates to greater use of social support and meeting the needs of others.

As discussed previously, the independent and autonomous self (high in personal agency) is more common and representative in Western, European, and American cultures where the self is seen as the source of individual action and success. The interconnected self (communal mastery) is more representative of Eastern Confucian-based cultures, such as China, Korea, and Japan (Hobfoll, Schroder, Wells, and Malek, 2002). From this perspective, individuals are understood in terms of their interconnectedness and attachments with others, and significant relationships with the family, workplace, and nation. Women in all cultures studied are more likely than men to see themselves as interconnected with others, and tend to see their actions as socially interwoven.

Consistent with theory, Asian Americans and Asians in Japan, South Korea, China, and India report lower levels of perceived control than non-Asians (Thompson, 2002). Compared with individualistic Western cultures, Asian cultures emphasize selfless subordination to family and community, which may decrease levels of personal control. In fact, high levels of personal control among Asians may be a violation of the norm, and individuals who pursue individual autonomy and personal goals may be punished. On the other hand, personal control has less impact on psychological distress for Asians, and may be associated less strongly with psychological well-being (Sastry & Ross, 1998). However, punishment for pursuing personal control would be expected to result in psychological distress.

Family decision-making has been found to be more significant than individual autonomy in studies done in Spain, France, Japan, and Eastern Europe. The decision-making styles of Mexican Americans, Korean Americans, and the Chinese are also family interdependent (Elliott, 2001). Black Americans have a lower sense of personal control than whites (Sastry & Ross, 1998).

Religion also affects sources of perceived control. Bangladeshi diabetics consider the dietary restrictions of Islam to be more important than those prescribed by doctors. Hindus regard cultural rules with respect to social roles and obligations to be important, even when they may be detrimental to health. For Hindus, who form the religious majority in India, control is not considered possible or even desirable, as it is in Western societies. Adherents to behaviorally strict religions, such as Mormons, have demonstrated the highest internal locus of control scores, whereas Presbyterians, whose religion emphasizes reverence to powerful church leaders, have had the highest powerful others (external locus of control) scores (Wrightson & Wardle, 1997).

INTERVENTIONS

Personal control is one of the most important factors determining whether or not an individual can alter self-defeating habits (Peterson & Stunkard, 1989). In fact, control may be a mediating factor in behavior change. The mastery of behaviors needed to reduce one risk factor may enhance an individual's personal control over other related behaviors. Motivation may be general, but beliefs are always specific.

Consequently, nursing interventions to enhance primary, internal, and personal control might include:

1. Teaching stress reduction and coping skills, especially those matched to the desired level of control.
2. Enhancing control by modeling behavior, encouraging the client to participate more in treatment decisions, positive self-talk, and identifying controllable and uncontrollable life events (Lazarus & Folkman, 1984).
3. Helping clients to help themselves by encouraging self-reliance, autonomy, and empowerment.
4. Fostering trust, praising positive behavior, encouraging choice, and affirming the clients' perspective.
5. Implementing models of service delivery that "emphasize self-reliance and autonomy, promote supportive environments, enhance access to user-friendly healthcare information, and address the needs of informal support networks" (Forbes, 2001, p. 32).

References

Antonovsky, A. (1987). *Unraveling the mystery of health: How people manage stress and stay well.* San Francisco: Jossey-Bass.

Cameron, L. D., & Leventhal, H. (2003). Self-regulation, health and illness. In L. D. Cameron & H. Leventhal (Eds.), *The self-regulation of health and illness behavior,* (pp. 1–13). London: Routledge.

Clark-Plaskie, M., & Lachman, M. E. (1999). The sense of control in mid-life. In S. L. Willis & J. D. Reid (Eds.), *Life in the middle: Psychological and social development in middle age* (pp. 182–208). San Diego, CA: Academic Press.

Davis, C. G., Nolen-Hoeksema, S., & Larson, J. (1998). Making sense of loss and benefiting from the experience: Two construals of meaning. *Journal of Personality and Social Psychology, 75,* 561–574.

Deci, E. L., & Ryan, R. M. (1985). *Intrinsic motivation and self-determination in human behavior.* New York: Plenum Press.

Elliott, A. C. (2001). Health care ethics: Cultural relativity of autonomy. *Journal of Transcultural Nursing, 12,* 326–330.

Folkman, S., & Moskowitz, J. T. (2000). Positive affect and the other side of coping. *American Psychologist, 55,* 647–654.

Forbes, E. A. (2001). Enhancing mastery and sense of coherence: Important determinants of health in older adults. *Geriatric Nursing, 22,* 29–32.

Fournier, G., & Jeanrie, C. (2003). Locus of control. In S. J. Lopez & C. R. Snyder (Eds.), *Positive psychological assessment: A handbook of models and measures* (pp. 139–154). Washington DC: American Psychological Association.

Fredrickson, B. L. (2001). The role of positive emotions in positive psychology: The broaden-and-build theory of positive emotions. *American Psychologist, 56,* 218–226.

Grob, A. (2000). Perceived control and subjective well-being across nations and across the life span. In E. Diener, & E. M. Suh (Eds.), *Culture and subjective well-being* (pp. 319–339). Cambridge MA: MIT Press.

Hobfoll, S. E., Schroder, K. E. E., Wells, M., & Malek, M. (2002). Communal versus individualistic construction of sense of mastery in facing life challenges. *Journal of Social and Clinical Psychology, 21,* 362–399.

Korotkov, D. (1998). The sense of coherence: Making sense out of chaos. In P. T. P. Wong & P. S. Fry (Eds.), *The human quest for meaning* (pp. 51–70). Mahwah, NJ: Lawrence Erlbaum.

Larsen, J. T., Hemenover, S. H., Norris, C. J., & Cacioppo, J. T. (2003). Turning adversity to advantage: On the virtues of the coactivation of positive and negative emotions. In L. G. Aspinwall & U. M. Steudinger (Eds.), *A psychology of human strengths. Fundamental questions and future directions for a positive psychology* (pp. 211–225). Washington DC: American Psychological Association.

Lazarus, R. S. (2003a). Does the positive psychology movement have legs? *Psychological Inquiry, 14,* 93–109.

Lazarus, R. S. (2003b). The Lazarus manifesto for positive psychology and psychology in general. *Psychological Inquiry, 14,* 173–189.

Lazarus, R. S., & Folkman, S. (1984). *Stress, appraisal and coping.* New York: Springer.

Moes, S., & Gebhardt, W. (2000). Self-regulation and health behavior: The health behavior goal model. In M. Boekaerts, P. R. Pintrich, & M. Zeidner (Eds.), *Handbook of self-regulation* (pp. 343–368). San Diego, CA: Academic Press.

Neuman, B. (2002). The Neuman systems model. In B. Neuman & J. Fawcett (Eds.), *The Neuman systems model* (4th ed.). Upper Saddle River, NJ: Prentice-Hall.

Park, C. L., & Folkman, S. (1998). Meaning in the context of stress and coping. *Review of General Psychology, 1,* 115–144.

Pearlin. L. I., & Pioli, M. F. (2003). Personal control: Some conceptual turf and future directions. In S. H. Zarit, L. J. Pearlin, & K. W. Schaie (Eds.), *Personal control in social and life course contexts* (pp. 1–21). New York: Springer.

Peterson, C. (1999). Personal control and well-being. In D. Kahnerman, E. Diener, & N. Schwartz (Eds.), *Well-being: The foundations of hedonic psychology* (pp. 288–301). Washington DC: American Psychological Association.

Peterson, C., & Stunkard, A. J. (1989). Personal control and health promotion. *Social Science and Medicine, 28,* 819–828.

Rodin, J. (1990). Control by any other name: Definitions, concepts, and processes. In J. Rodin, C. Schooler, & K. W. Schaie (Eds.), *Self-directedness: Cause and effects throughout the life course* (pp. 1–17). Hillsdale, NJ: Lawrence Erlbaum.

Ross, C. E., & Sastry, J. (1999). The sense of personal control: Social-structural causes and emotional consequences. In C. A. Aneshensel & J. C. Phelan (Eds.), *Handbook of the sociology of mental health* (pp. 369–394). New York: Kluwer Academic/Plenum.

Rotter, J. B. (1966). Generalized expectancies for internal vs. external control of reinforcements. *Psychological Monographs, 80,* 1–28.

Ryan, R. M. (1982). Control and information in the intrapersonal sphere: An extension of cognitive evaluation theory. *Journal of Personality and Social Psychology, 43,* 450–461.

Sastry, J., & Ross, C. E. (1998). Asian ethnicity and the sense of personal control. *Social Psychology Quarterly, 61,* 101–120.

Schwarzer, R., & Knoll, N. (2003). Positive coping: Mastering demands and searching for meaning. In S. J. Lopez, & C. R. Snyder (Eds.), *Positive psychological assessment: A handbook of models and measures* (pp. 393–409). Washington DC: American Psychological Association.

Skaff, M. M., & Gardiner, P. (2003). Cultural variations in the meaning of control. In S. H. Zarit, L. J. Pearlin, & K. W. Schaie (Eds.), *Personal control in social and life course contexts* (pp. 83–105). New York: Springer.

Skinner, E. A. (1996). A guide to constructs of control. *Journal of Personality and Social Psychology, 71,* 549–570.

Somerfield, M. R., & McCrae, R. R. (2003). Stress and coping research: Methodological challenges, theoretical advances, and clinical applications. *American Psychologist, 55,* 620–625.

Syme, S. L. (1990). Control and health: An epidemiological perspective. In J. Rodin, C. Schooler, & K. W. Schaie (Eds.), *Self-directedness: Cause and effects throughout the life course* (pp. 213–229). Hillsdale, NJ: Lawrence Erlbaum.

Thompson, S. C. (2002). The role of personal control in adaptive functioning. In C. R. Snyder & S. J. Lopez (Eds.), *Handbook of positive psychology* (pp. 202–213). Oxford: Oxford University Press.

Weise, J. R. (1990). Development of control-related beliefs, goals, and styles in childhood and adolescence: A clinical perspective. In J. Rodin, C. Schooler, & K. W. Schaie (Eds.), *Self-directedness: Cause and effects throughout the life course* (pp. 103–145). Hillsdale, NJ: Lawrence Erlbaum.

Wrightson, K. J., & Wardle, J. (1997). Cultural variation in health locus of control. *Ethnicity and Health, 2,* 13–20 (retrieved electronically).

Zimmerman, B. J. (2000). Attaining self-regulation: A social cognitive perspective. In M. Boekaerts, P. R. Pintrich, & M. Zeidner (Eds.), *Handbook of self-regulation* (pp. 13–39). San Diego, CA: Academic Press.

CHAPTER 8

Power Part Three: Choice

Concepts
Creativity
Self-Determination

Models and Theories
Rogers' Science of Unitary Human
 Beings

Self-Determination Model of
 Well-Being

Helpful Lists
Interventions to Facilitate Choice,
 pg. 109

Thought Questions
1. What is the difference between freedom to and freedom from?
2. How do freedom and alternatives affect choice?
3. What are signature characteristics of creativity? How can creativity be stimulated?
4. How are flexibility and self-determination related?
5. Describe interventions you can use to generate client choices.

Chapter Synopsis
This chapter introduces the concept of choice as a human strength as a resource for health. Choice is closely related to the Healthiness Theory concepts of goals, challenge, capability, control, capacity, confidence, and connection. Rogers' nursing model, the Science of Unitary Human Beings, is discussed briefly. The related concepts of creativity and self-determination are differentiated from choice. Finally, intervention strategies to increase alternatives for choice are presented.

CHOICE

Choice means more than just making conscious decisions. Choice is motivational whereas decision-making is cognitive. Choice involves freedom and refers to the extent an individual "is his own master," regarding decisions that are not influenced by external forces or circumstances. "Freedom is quintessentially concerned with the absence of restraint and interference by others" (Sen, 1988, p. 273). Freedom should allow choice. A lack of freedom can be considered a deprivation of power.

Choice is a freedom *to* rather than freedom *from*, and involves noninterference, meaning that constraints are not imposed on individuals as they exercise their liberty. The individual must make a voluntary, intuitive, and spontaneous choice free from undue influence or coercion. Freedom is not a property, or something an individual possesses, but a relationship between agents (Bavetia & DelSeta, 2001).

An individual's independent decisions depend on the number of alternatives from which to choose. Greater freedom of choice designates "an increased flexibility, a widened spectrum of possible responses to inner and outer stimuli, and an expanded universe of psychological possibilities" (Abend, 2001, p. 3). Thus, freedom is viewed as having a variety of unrestricted choices (freedom from constraints) (Bavetia & DelSeta, 2001). Having different opportunities available reflects a certain degree of freedom.

The value of choice is that it will lead to something (Suzuki, 2002). "Choice is not just about being able to choose between a bottle of wine and a banana. It is rather about one's choice of what bottle of wine to buy being totally unrestricted and autonomous" (Bavetia & DelSeta, 2001, p. 220). However, freedom may be inhibited if the choices and alternatives are too similar. Having more alternatives leads to more selective and stronger preferences, and provides more opportunities for creativity. Choice is assumed to go in the direction of the alternative that seems to be most attractive.

For example, in a multichoice task, students' preference for an alternative depended on opportunity of choice, reinforcement, efficacy (effectiveness) of choice, and the number of alternatives. In a meta-analysis of 13 studies with 30 primarily adolescent participants, it was determined that providing choices resulted in a clinically significant reduction in the number of occurrences of problem behavior (Shogren, Faggella-Luby, Bae, and Wehmeyer, 2004). However, when options cannot be differentiated (one option is not better than another), choice does not seem to be very significant. When individuals accommodate to available choices they gain a realistic sense of what is possible (Deci & Ryan, 1985). The ability to accept a particular situation is a good predictor of well-being.

In a study testing the relationship between choice and quality of life among residents in long-term care facilities, a significant positive correlation was found between the amount of choice residents felt they had and their quality of life (Duncan-Myers & Huebner, 2000). In other words, more choices resulted in patients feeling better about their quality of life. Programs that empowered residents to make small, everyday choices helped to improve their health, quality of life, and life satisfaction. Choice-making was one way to improve an internal locus of control and enhance a sense of control. This concept can be applied in the client-nurse relationship by helping clients discover opportunities to make choices, even if the choices are minor. This might mean allowing clients to choose the time of a test or treatment, which foods to add to a special diet, or which arm should be used for an intravenous infusion. Having choice gives clients a sense of control.

VALUES AND CHOICE BETWEEN ALTERNATIVES

Values are the beliefs that individuals have about desirable ways of behaving or about desirable end states (Feather, 1995). There is an "oughtness" about them. Values are relatively stable (although not unchanging), function as criteria or frameworks against which experience can be tested, are more abstract than attitudes, and are hierarchically organized in their importance (Feather, 1995).

"Values [also] have long-term motivational effects on a person's behavior, functioning to influence both short-term and long-term goals and the selection of plans and actions that relate to these goals" (Feather, 1995). For example, research has demonstrated that after making a choice, Americans justify the choice to eliminate doubts about their capability, whereas the Japanese justify their choice to gain the positive appraisal of others (Kitayama, Suibbe, Markus, and Suzuki, 2004). In contrast, attitudes maintain some stability across a wider time frame, and can function as motives, like needs, to influence goal-directed behavior.

CHOICE-RELATED MODEL

Rogers' Science of Unitary Human Beings

Rogers' science is a nursing model that emphasizes the fostering of health potential as the purpose of nursing. Individuals are active participants in the search for health. Therefore they seek choices in order to grow within constant change. Rogers proposes three principles to explain the evolution of the life process and to describe aspects of change: integrality, helicy, and resonancy. The principle of integrality emphasizes that the human energy field and the environmental energy field are continuous and must be perceived simultaneously. There is no cause and effect, but rather mutual process through a web of interrelationships. The principle of helicy predicts that change occurs as a "continuous innovative, unpredictable, increasing diversity of human and environmental field patterns" (Rogers, 1990, p. 8). Choices are essential to innovation and for participation in changes that promote increasing diversity. The principle of resonancy indicates that change in pattern toward increased complexity occurs by way of waves "manifesting continuous change from lower frequency, longer wave patterns to higher frequency, shorter wave pattern" (Rogers, 1980, p. 333). This principle is consistent with Leddy's Energy-Based Practice Theory (see Chapter 11). Both Rogers and Leddy believe that it is possible to intervene by using awareness and choice to affect client patterning.

RELATED CONCEPTS

Creativity

Creativity has been defined as "the ability of individuals and groups to produce novel ideas that are useful and appropriate to a given situation" (Grawitch, Munz, Elliott, and Mathis, 2003, p. 201). Creativity develops useful or influential original ideas (Runco, 2004). As a consequence, creative solutions to a problem possess novelty, uniqueness, or originality. Creativity can be evaluated on the absolute number of ideas (fluency); variety of ideas (flexibility); unusualness of the ideas (originality); and/or the ability to build on other ideas (elaboration) (Grawitch et al., 2003).

Creative ideas allow the individual to remain flexible, facilitating growth and late-life adaptation. Creative individuals value art and beauty, have broad interests, are attracted to complexity, have high energy, are able to make independent judgments, are autonomous, intuitive, self-confident, have an ability to resolve conflicts, and can accommodate apparently conflicting traits in their self-concept, and finally, have a firm sense of self as "creative" (Runco, 2004). They tend to follow intrinsic interests and see time as an important resource essential to creative insight. They view creative insight as a long drawn out thought process and not a quick "aha" moment. Creativity contributes to optimal functioning and "facilitates and enhances problem solving, adaptability, self-expression, and health" (Runco, 2004, p. 677).

Influences that stimulate creativity include freedom, autonomy, good role models and resources (including time), encouragement specifically for originality, freedom from criticism, and norms that prize innovation and do not consider failure a disaster. Some influences can also inhibit creativity. These include a lack of respect (specifically for originality), red tape, constraint, lack of autonomy and resources, inappropriate norms, project management, feedback, time pressure, competition, and unrealistic expectations (Runco, 2004). Environments that support creativity allow independent work, are stimulating but not distracting, and provide easy assess to resources. Originality is the most widely acknowledged requisite for creativity. But originality alone is not sufficient for creativity.

Behavioral correlates of creativity include insight and novelty. Experience can increase the likelihood of insights. Creativity reflects originality and appropriateness, intuition, and logic, and requires the capacities from both hemispheres of the brain. Associative or connective processes can contribute to creative thinking and problem-solving. However, although creativity can facilitate problem-solving, not all creativity involves problem-solving, and not all problem-solving requires creativity. Key cognitive aspects of creativity include conceptualization, imagination, expansive attention for discovering remote and original ideas, incubation, insight, intuition, simultaneous consideration of two very different perspectives, logic, metaphors, mindfulness, misjudgment, and perspective.

The Self-Determination Model of Well-Being

The self-determination model of well-being proposes that there are three universal psychological needs, autonomy, competence, and relatedness. The key predictor of an individual's psychological well-being is whether these needs are met. This model predicts that pursing intrinsic goals provides individuals with a deep sense of satisfaction, whereas pursuing extrinsic goals do not. In other words, according to the self-determination theory, the 'good life' is "the life in which an individual strives for personal growth, independence, meaningful relationships with others, and community service" (Oishi, 2000, pp. 87–88).

Self-determination is the capacity to freely choose apart from undue external influence or interference (Deci & Ryan, 1985; Schalock & Alonso, 2002) such as reinforcements, drives, forces, or pressures. Rewards, widely used as instruments of control, can often co-opt or diminish self-determination, stimulating different motivational dynamics. For example, when a child is offered a treat to get ready for school, the reward (the treat) becomes the motivation for behavior, rather than feeling of pride for meeting a goal.

Self-determination is more than a capacity, it is also a need. Individuals who are self-determined make things happen in their lives, they are causal agents. However, causal agency implies action that is intended to accomplish a specific end, rather than just making something happen (action for the sake of action). Causal agency and its actions are designed to improve the individual's quality of life. The degree to which an individual is self-determined either influences or is influenced by other core dimensions of overall (global) quality of life (Schalock & Alonso, 2002).

The psychological hallmark of self-determination is flexibility in managing both the self and the environment. The individual must have control over outcomes because being unable to control outcomes (which precludes self-determination), has negative consequences. Essential characteristics of self-determined behavior include: behavioral autonomy and interdependence; self-regulated behavior; acting in a psychologically empowered manner, with efficacy, locus of control, and motivation; and self-realization.

INTERVENTIONS

Following are some interventions nurses can use to help clients generate choices (Nezu, Nazu, Friedman, Faddis, and Houts, 1998). In this case, quantity breeds quality, so it is important to write down as many choices and alternatives as possible.

1. Defer judgment about choices—generate as many choices as possible.
2. Use strategies and tactics—encourage general courses of action rather than specific steps—don't get bogged down with details.
3. Stay focused—avoid getting sidetracked by multiple alternatives.
4. Combine ideas—if this is possible, the ideas can be retained without unnecessary proliferation of choices.
5. Modify existing alternatives—this can be an excellent source of ideas to supplement brainstorming of new alternatives.
6. Use models and heroes (exemplars)—a framework can suggest multiple alternatives.
7. Apply visualization techniques—by imagining and picturing alternatives, it may be possible to gain added clarity and detail.

References
Abend, S. M. (2001). Expanding psychological possibilities. *Psychoanalytic quarterly, 70,* 3–14.
Bavetia, S., & DelSeta, M. (2001). Constraints and the measurement of freedom of choice. *Theory and Decision, 50,* 213–238.
Deci, E. L., & Ryan, R. M. (1985). *Intrinsic motivation and self-determination in human behavior.* New York: Plenum Press.
Duncan-Myers, A. M., & Huebner, R. A. (2000). Relationship between choice and quality of life among residents in long-term care facilities. *American Journal of Occupational Therapy, 54,* 504–508.
Feather, N. T. (1995). Values, valences, and choice: The influence of values on the perceived attractiveness and choice of alternatives. *Journal of Personality and Social Psychology, 68,* 1135–1151.
Grawitch, M. J., Munz, D. C., Elliott, E. K., & Mathis, A. (2003). Promoting creativity in temporary problem-solving groups: The effects of positive mood and autonomy in problem definition on idea-generating performance. *Group Dynamics: Theory, Research and Practice, 7,* 200–213.
Kitayama, S., Suibbe, A. C., Markus, H. R., & Suzuki, T. (2004). Is there any "free" choice? Self and dissonance in two cultures. *Psychological Science, 15,* 527–533.

Nezu, A. M., Nazu, C. M., Friedman, S. H., Faddis, S., & Houts, P. S. (1998). *Helping cancer patients cope: A problem-solving approach.* Washington DC: American Psychological Association.

Oishi, S. (2000). Goals as cornerstones of subjective well-being: Linking individuals and cultures. In E. Diener & E. M. Suh (Eds.), *Culture and subjective well-being* (pp. 87–112). Cambridge, MA: MIT Press.

Rogers, M. E. (1980). Nursing: A science of unitary man. In J. P. Riehl & C. Roy (Eds.), *Conceptual models for nursing practice* (pp. 329–337). New York: Appleton-Century-Crofts.

Rogers, M. E. (1990). Nursing: Science of unitary irreducible human beings: Update 1990. In E. A. M. Barrett (Ed.), *Visions of Rogers' science based nursing* (pp. 5–11). New York: National League for Nursing.

Runco, M. A. (2004). Creativity. *Annual Review of Psychology, 55,* 657–687.

Schalock, R. L., & Alonso, M. A. V. (2002*). Handbook on quality of life for human service practitioners.* Washington DC: American Association on Mental Retardation.

Sen, A. (1988). Freedom of choice. *European Economic Review, 32,* 269–294.

Shogren, K. A., Faggella-Luby, M. N., Bae, S. J., & Wehmeyer, M. L. (2004). The effect of choice-making as an intervention for problem behavior. *Journal of Positive Behavior Interventions, 6,* 228–237.

Suzuki, S. (2002). Preference for freedom of choice. In S. P. Shohov (Ed.), *Advances in psychology research, vol 9* (pp. 115–128).

CHAPTER 9

Power Part Four: Challenge

Concepts
Resilience
Flow
Proactive Coping
Humor

Theory
Newman's Theory of Health as
   Expanding Consciousness

Helpful Lists
Challenge and Opportunities for
   Success, pgs. 112–113
Characteristics of Flow, pg. 114
Stages of Proactive Coping, pg. 115
Benefits of Proactive Coping, pg. 115

Thought Questions
1. Compare challenge viewed from a threat-avoidant coping perspective versus a strengths perspective.
2. Describe flow. How does flow relate to strengths concepts such as challenge, control, and goals?
3. How is proactive coping different from threat-avoidant coping? Why is this difference important for nurses to understand?
4. How can you promote proactive coping in practice?

Chapter Synopsis
This chapter introduces the concept of challenge as a human strength as a resource for health. Challenge is closely related to the Healthiness Theory concepts of meaning, goals, choice, confidence, and control. Newman's Theory of Health as Expanding Consciousness is discussed. Related concepts, such as proactive coping, resilience, flow, and humor, are differentiated from challenge.

CHALLENGE

In the literature, challenge is referred to exclusively within the context of stress and coping. Stress is relational in nature, arising from a transaction between the individual and the environment. Stress is a judgment that particular demands of a situation exceed the resources for dealing with them, which directly affects the individual's sense of well-being. Individuals initially evaluate what is at stake through a primary appraisal and then, through secondary appraisal, gauge the controllability of the situation. When a situation is seen as an opportunity for self-growth and coping strategies are available to manage the demands identified, stress is perceived in terms of challenge (Drach-Zahavy & Erez, 2002).

A disposition toward challenge is the belief that change (rather than stability) is normal in life and that change is an interesting incentive to growth rather than threatening to security (Kobasa, Maddi, and Kahn, 1982). Challenge occurs when the environmental demands and goals of a situation fit with the individual's resources and ability to cope. A challenge response is associated with a positive affect or low negative affect and efficient or organized mobilization of physiological resources (Tomaka, Blascovich, Kibler, and Ernst, 1997). Feeling positive about a demanding encounter is a hallmark of feeling challenged (Lazarus & Folkman, 1984) and is reflected in the pleasurable emotions accompanying challenge. "Challenge is experienced when there is an opportunity for self-growth with available coping strategies" (Drach-Zahavy & Erez, 2002, p. 667).

Cognitive appraisal processes automatically intervene between the initial perception and subsequent experience of a potentially stressful situation (Tomaka, Blascovich, Kelsey, and Leitten, 1993). Challenge leads to self transformation and growth rather than to conserving and protecting the past (Kobasa et al., 1982). Individuals who are challenged are more confident, less emotionally overwhelmed, and more capable of drawing on available resources than individuals who are inhibited or blocked by their response to an appraised threat (Lazarus & Folkman, 1984, p. 34). Challenge appraisals focus on the potential for gain or growth and are characterized by pleasurable emotions, such as eagerness, excitement and exhilaration. In contrast, changes that are viewed as threats rather than challenges focus on potential harm and are characterized by negative emotions, such as fear, anxiety, and anger. The perception of inequalities and that life has been unfair, including having a lower socioeconomic status, decrease the odds of having positive psychological outcomes when facing challenges.

An individual who strives to accomplish difficult goals when task complexity is high, may perceive the goal as a challenge rather than a threat, resulting in higher levels of performance (Drach-Zahavy & Erez, 2002). Complex tasks consist of *component* complexity (number of performance components), such as acts to perform, *coordinating* complexity (coordination required to complete the task), and *dynamic* complexity (changes in the predictability of acts and information cues). Effective performance of complex tasks depends on the amount of effort exerted in the task, and the development of relevant strategies. A challenge entails stretching personal abilities in order to try something new, with enjoyment and excitement as the rewards (Deci & Ryan, 1985).

Threat and challenge may be viewed as dimensions of the same rhythmical pattern and not necessarily as opposite poles of a single continuum. Thus, they may not be mutually exclusive (Lazarus & Folkman, 1984). Challenge and threat appraisals result in distinct (e.g., problem/emotion-focused, or active/passive) patterns of coping, with challenge leading to a vigilant ("on guard") coping pattern. Associations have been found between challenge and opportunities for success including:

- Social rewards, such as recognition and praise, mastery, learning, and personal growth (Skinner & Brewer, 2002)

- Positive emotions, such as happiness and hope
- Expectations of favorable performance, certainty of performance level, perceptions of increased control, and anticipation of effort
- Hope-challenge emotions and perceptions of high problem-focused coping opportunities and optimistic expectations
- Challenge emotions and appraisals of effort and interest, such as feeling confident, hopeful, or eager (Skinner & Brewer, 2002)

Challenge appraisals are more likely to occur when the individual has a sense of control within the human-environment relationship. But challenge only occurs if what must be done calls for substantial efforts. "The joy of challenge is that one pits oneself against the odds" (Lazarus & Folkman, 1984, p. 36). Challenge can also be defined as exerting self-control in the face of adversity, and overcoming adversity rather than feeling helpless (Lazarus & Folkman, 1984). When individuals feel threatened they see potential loss with little to be gained, whereas those who are challenged see the possibility of gain.

Challenge is inversely related to negative emotional reactions, and positively related to physiological activity. In other words, challenge decreases negative emotions and increases physiological activity. Physiological activation in response to challenge is related primarily to energy mobilization and effort (Tomaka et al., 1993). Cardiac reactivity during active coping has been related positively to challenge appraisals and negatively to threat appraisals. Conversely, vascular reactivity has been related positively to threat appraisals and negatively to challenge appraisals. Thus, challenge can have a direct effect on physiology in general and specifically on cardiac and vascular activity. Challenge seems to increase both perceived and actual performance during active coping (Tomaka et al., 1993).

When individuals are presented a task, where objective evaluation is not emphasized, and are encouraged to do their best, challenge-related appraisals and physiology can result (Tomaka et al., 1997). When the work context is perceived as challenging, a difficult goal can induce high adaptation to change (Drach-Zahavy & Erez, 2002). When comparing threat appraisals to trait (enduring personality characteristics) and state (brief context-related) challenge appraisals, it was discovered that challenge tends to result in confident coping expectancies, lower perceptions of threat, higher positive emotions, and more beneficial effects on emotion and performance than threat appraisals (Skinner & Brewer, 2002).

THEORY

Newman's Theory of Health as Expanding Consciousness

Newman's nursing theory of Health as Expanding Consciousness views health as a process that encompasses both disease and "nondisease." Instead of the familiar linear relationship between health as good and disease or illness as bad, Newman conceptualizes disease as a meaningful component of the whole individual and a possible facilitator of health. Consciousness is expressed in patterns of rhythmic movement toward higher levels. Manifestations of these patterns include exchanging, communicating, relating, valuing, choosing, moving, perceiving, feeling, and knowing, all actions that are relevant to challenge. Nursing facilitates the process of evolving to higher levels of consciousness by "rhythmic connecting of the nurse with the client in an authentic way for the purpose of illuminating the pattern and discovering the new rules of a higher level of organization" (Newman, 1990, p. 40).

RELATED CONCEPTS

Resilience

Resilience is "the capacity to prevail in the face of adversity… the maintenance, recovery, or improvement to mental or physical health following challenge" (Ryff & Singer, 2003, p. 20). Frequently, resilience is related to thriving after a traumatic experience. In fact, resilience has been associated with such outcomes as sense of coherence, hardiness, toughening, feeling like a survivor rather than victim, increased self-reliance and self-efficacy, increased awareness of vulnerability and mortality, improvement in ties to others (increased self-disclosure and emotional expressiveness, increased compassion and capacity to give to others, a clearer philosophy of life), a renewed sense of priorities and appreciation of life, and a deeper sense of meaning and spirituality (Ryff & Singer, 2003).

Resilience is an adaptive response to immediate threats (stressors) with the goal of restoring equilibrium. Resilience should be considered a consequence of challenge. In contrast, positive events or experiences provide resources for health and growth in the near- or long-term. It should be clear that resilience (response to threats) is conceptualized quite differently from growth-promoting resources (responses to positive events). It is important to distinguish between maintenance and restoration from a negative perspective (e.g., resilience, with an unattainable goal of stability), and growth and development from a positive perspective (e.g., flow, with the potential of achieving harmony and self-actualization).

Flow

Flow is characterized by complete absorption in a task (Nakamura & Csikszentmihalyi, 2002). Flow includes challenges or opportunities for action that stretch existing skills but do not overextend or underutilize them. A sense of engaging in challenges appropriate to individual capacities is also present. Flow provides clear immediate goals and feedback about progress. It is an intrinsically motivated activity that is rewarding in and of itself apart from the end product. Two kinds of experiences can be intrinsically rewarding: one involving conservation of energy (relaxation), the other involving the use of skills to seize ever-greater opportunities (flow).

Characteristics of flow include:

- Intense and focused concentration on the present task
- Merging of action and awareness
- Losing reflective self-awareness
- A sense of self-control
- Time passing more quickly
- Experiencing an activity as intrinsically rewarding, so that the end goal is just an excuse for the process (Nakamura & Csikszentmihalyi, 2002)

Flow is a subjective state, balanced between capacities and opportunities. "If challenges begin to exceed skills, one first becomes vigilant and then anxious; if skills begin to exceed changes, first one relaxes and then becomes bored" (Nakamura & Csikszentmihalyi, 2002, p. 90). Flow contributes to quality of life by providing momentary experiences with value, and it can buffer adversity and prevent pathology.

Proactive Coping

"Coping is defined as the process of managing internal or external demands that are appraised as taxing or exceeding the resources of a person" (Lazarus & Folkman, 1984). Proactive coping involves taking actions to prevent or modify a potentially stressful event before it occurs (Aspinwall & Taylor, 1997). Proactive coping occurs before anticipatory coping. It involves building and accumulating resources and skills, not to deal with a spe-cific anticipated stressor, but to prepare in general. Available resources play a critical role (not a moderating role) in whether a stressor is experienced, what form it will take, and how fully developed it is when it must be dealt with (Aspinwall & Taylor, 1997). Effective proactive coping, which is virtually always active, involves the mustering of time, money, planning and organizational skills, and social support.

Nurses can encourage clients to practice coping, by understanding the five stages of proactive coping described by Aspinwall & Taylor (1997):

1. *Resource accumulation*—building resources and skills in advance of any specific anticipated stressor.
2. *Recognition*—being able to see a potential stressful event coming. This depends on being able to screen the environment for danger and being sensitive to internal cues suggesting that threats may arise.
3. *Initial appraisal*—detecting the stressor, and assessing the current (What is this?) and potential (What is this likely to become?) status of the potential stressor.
4. *Initial coping efforts*—taking action (rather than avoiding) to prevent or minimize a recognized or suspected stressor.
5. *Elicitation and use of feedback*—acquiring and using feedback about the stressful event and the success of preliminary coping efforts, and evaluating whether the stressor requires additional coping efforts. This is the final step in the proactive coping process.

Benefits of proactive coping (Aspinwall & Taylor, 1997) include:

1. Focusing on the future rather than trying to compensate for loss or harm in the past
2. Being goal oriented, resulting in difficult situations being perceived as challenges
3. Being positively motivated, finding challenge stimulating, resulting in general resources being built up to support goals and personal growth
4. Lower levels of stress experienced during a stressful encounter
5. Tackling the stressor in its early stages, when the ratio of coping resources to the magnitude of a stressor is likely to be more favorable
6. Anticipating a stressful event, resulting in having more options available to manage it

Active coping is superior to avoidant coping. Active behavioral coping is consistently associated with positive emotional adjustment. Differences that predispose individuals toward active coping in controllable situations also appear to promote emotion-focused coping for uncontrollable stressors. To the extent that proactive coping enables individuals to prevent, offset, eliminate, reduce, or modify impending stressful events, proactive coping eliminates much stress before it occurs (Aspinwall & Taylor, 1997). Several strategies that professional caregivers can use to aid proactive coping include providing relevant information and effective support, and helping clients to reframe experiences and infuse ordinary events with positive meaning.

Humor

"Sense of humor may be conceptualized as a habitual behavior pattern, such as a tendency to laugh frequently, to tell jokes and amuse others, to 'get the joke,' or to remember jokes; a temperamental trait of habitual cheerfulness; an aesthetic response such as enjoyment of a particular type of humorous material; a positive attitude toward humor and humorous people; a bemused outlook on life, or a coping strategy of having a tendency to maintain a humorous perspective in the face of adversity. Humor is not wit, comedy, sarcasm, irony, satire, or ridicule... Humor is a sympathetic, tolerant, and benevolent amusement at the imperfections of the world and the foibles of human nature in general" (Martin, 2003, pp. 313–314). Individuals with a humorous outlook are self-deprecating yet self-accepting, are characterized by chuckling rather than hearty laughter; do not take themselves too seriously; are able to poke fun at themselves; and maintain a philosophical detachment from adversity.

Coping with stress involves a cognitive process of appraising potentially stressful situations in a more benign, less threatening manner (Martin, 2003). Those individuals with a good sense of humor have increased social support, are more extroverted, and get along well with others; and have better health and are better able to cope with stress (Martin, 2003).

References

Aspinwall, L. G., & Taylor, S. E. (1997). A stitch in time: Self-regulation and proactive coping. *Psychological Bulletin, 121,* 417–436.

Deci, E. L., & Ryan, R. M. (1985). *Intrinsic motivation and self-determination in human behavior.* New York: Plenum Press.

Drach-Zahavy, A., & Erez, M. (2002). Challenge versus threat effects on the goal-performance relationship. *Organizational Behavior and Human Decision Processes, 88,* 667–682.

Kobasa, S. C., Maddi, S. R., & Kahn, S. (1982). Hardiness and health: A perspective study. *Journal of Personality and Social Psychology, 42,* 168–177.

Lazarus, R. S., & Folkman, S. (1984). *Stress, appraisal and coping.* New York: Springer.

Martin, R. (2003). Sense of humor. In S. J. Lopez & C. R. Snyder (Eds.), *Positive psychological assessment. A handbook of models and methods* (pp. 313–326). Washington DC: American Psychological Association.

Nakamura, J., & Csikszentmihalyi, M. (2002). The motivational sources of creativity as viewed from the paradigm of positive psychology. In L. G. Aspinwall & U. M. Steudinger (Eds.), *A psychology of human strengths. Fundamental questions and future directions for a positive psychology* (pp. 257–269). Washington DC: American Psychological Association.

Newman, M. A. (1990). Toward an integrative model of professional practice. *Journal of Professional Nursing, 6,* 167–173.

Ryff, C. D., & Singer, B. (2003). Thriving in the face of challenge: The integrative science of human resilience. In F. Kessel, P. L. Rosenfield, & N. B. Anderson (Eds.), *Expanding the boundaries of health and social science* (pp. 181–205). Oxford: Oxford University Press.

Skinner, N., & Brewer, N. (2002). The dynamics of threat and challenge appraisals prior to stressful achievement events. *Journal of Personality and Social Psychology, 83,* 678–692.

Tomaka, J., Blascovich, J., Kelsey, R. M., & Leitten, C. L. (1993). Subjective, physiological, and behavioral effects of threat and challenge appraisal. *Journal of Personality and Social Psychology, 65,* 248–260.

Tomaka, J., Blascovich, J., Kibler, J., & Ernst, J. M. (1997). Cognitive and physiological antecedents of threat and challenge appraisal. *Journal of Personality and Social Psychology, 73,* 63–72.

CHAPTER 10

Power Part Five: Confidence

Concepts
Self-Concept
Self-Esteem

Models and Theories
Roy's Adaptation Theory
Sociometer Theory
Schema Model of the Self-Concept
Bonham-Cheney Model of Self-Concept
Status Dynamic Approach to Self-
    Concept

Helpful Lists
Schema Assessment, pg. 124
Implications for Nursing Interventions,
    pgs. 124–125
Labels Associated with Self-Esteem,
    pg. 126
Cultural Norms for Behavior,
    pg. 126
Distorted Ideas about Self-Esteem,
    pg. 127
Countering Techniques, pg. 128

Thought Questions

1. Contrast confidence and capability. Why is it important to understand the difference?
2. Why is confidence important in a strengths context?
3. How do actual, possible, and working selves differ? What is important about these distinctions?
4. How do cultural norms affect perceptions of capability, self-esteem, and self-confidence?
5. How can you foster client perceptions of confidence in your nursing practice?

Chapter Synopsis

This chapter introduces the concept of confidence as a human strength and as a resource for health. Confidence is closely related to the Healthiness Theory concepts of goals, connection, choice, challenge, and capability. The related concepts of self-concept and self-esteem are differentiated from confidence. Roy's Adaptation Theory of nursing and the Sociometer Theory are described, and implications for multicultural competency are discussed. Finally, intervention strategies to promote confidence are presented.

CONFIDENCE

Confidence can be defined as a strong, generalized, positive belief or certainty that individuals have about who they are. Confidence is closely related to self-image and to the decision-making process that occurs before taking action (Kear, 2000). Consequently, in the literature, confidence is implicit in discussions of self-concept and self-esteem. Confidence is associated with sureness in belief about the self, and is an antecedent to control. In contrast, capability is associated with beliefs about being able to act in a specific context to accomplish a task. Confidence facilitates and may mediate capability and leads to increased persistence and perseverance toward goals.

Self-confidence helps to buffer performance anxiety. Hanton and colleagues (2004) found that when self-confidence is absent competitive anxiety intensifies and, when it is seen as out of the individual's control, performance is hindered. In contrast, when self-confidence is high, increases in symptoms associated with anxiety lead to positive perceptions of control and interpretations that support proactive coping. To protect against debilitating interpretations of competitive anxiety, participants in the study reported the use of cognitive management strategies including mental rehearsal, thought stopping, and positive self-talk.

MODELS AND THEORIES

Roy's Adaptation Model

The essence of Roy's nursing model is adaptive behaviors; the set of processes the individual uses to adapt to environmental stimuli. There are three types of stimuli: focal (a change that immediately confronts the individual and requires an adaptive response), contextual (all other stimuli present), and residual (other relevant factors, such as non-specific stimuli), which mediate and contribute to the effect of the stimulus. The pooled effect of the three classes of stimuli results in the individual's adaptation level. Individuals are conceptualized by Roy as having four adaptive modes, or categories of behavior resulting from coping: physiologic-physical, self-concept-group identity, role function, and interdependence. The desired end result is a state in which conditions promote the individual's goals, including survival, growth, reproduction, mastery, and personal and environmental transformations. The goal of nursing is "to promote adaptation by the use of the nursing process, in each of the adaptive modes, thus contributing to health, quality of life, and dying with dignity" (Roy, 1987, p. 43).

Sociometer Theory

The Sociometer Theory, as the name implies, is concerned with social acceptance. It is assumed that self-esteem is used to monitor the likelihood of social exclusion; individuals with high self-esteem do not worry about how others see them, but individuals with low self-esteem are highly motivated by social anxiety to manage their public impressions (Heatherton & Wyland, 2003).

All individuals have a fundamental need to belong. Belonging is defined as "the degree to which an individual believes that other people regard their relationships with him or her to be valuable or important" (Leary & MacDonald, 2003, p. 403). A sense of belongingness affects self-esteem and confidence and develops over time as a result of being accepted or rejected by others. Self-esteem does not cause responses, traits, or patterns of behavior, and does not necessarily reflect on an individual's true value, worth, or desirability. These behaviors and beliefs are all the result of real, imagined, or anticipated acceptance and rejection. According to the theory, perceived relational value mediates the individual's self-assessments of abilities and attributes and a personal sense of self-worth (Leary & MacDonald, 2003).

Individuals with confidence and high self-esteem feel good about themselves. They are able to cope effectively with challenges and negative feedback, and they live in a social world in which they believe they are valued and respected. In contrast, substantial evidence shows a link between low confidence and low self-esteem with depression, shyness, and loneliness (Heatherton & Wyland, 2003).

RELATED CONCEPTS

Self-Concept

Self-concept encompasses everything that is known about the self, the totality of the beliefs that individuals have about themselves (Heatherton & Wyland, 2003). "The self-concept is viewed as a cognitive schema that controls the processing of self-relevant information, and organizes abstract and concrete memories about the self" (Campbell, 1990, p. 539). The self orients, mediates, and interprets an individual's experience, shaping what individuals notice and think about, what they are motivated to do, and how they feel and their ways of feeling. It is the meaningfulness and significance of the entire individual considered from a particular point of view (Markus & Kitayama, 1994). Core self conceptions are accessible over time, and provide some stability of self-perception throughout an individual's lifespan.

The self is the part of each individual that they are consciously aware of (Seigley, 1999). Self-concept consists of a global, introspective, and composite description of what individuals believe about themselves, their interpretations of past experiences and expectations about the future, and feelings of self-worth (Jones, 2004). Therefore, the self-concept provides the individual with a sense of continuity in time and space by integrating and organizing experience, regulating moods, and providing incentives or motivation (Markus & Wurf, 1987). The self-concept "interprets and organizes self-relevant actions and experiences; it has motivational consequences, providing the incentives, standards, plans, rules, and scripts for behavior, and it adjusts in response to challenges from the social environment" (Markus & Wurf, 1987, pp. 299–300). Self-concept is descriptive and does not involve a value judgment (King, 1997). The self-concept also mediates and regulates ongoing behavior, enabling dynamic, active, forceful, change-producing self-enhancement, consistency maintenance, and self-actualization (Markus & Wurf, 1987).

Through self-regulation of behaviors each individual tries to maintain a positive self-concept in a world of dynamic interactions (Kear, 2000). According to Markus and Wurf

(1987) self-concept is viewed as a collection of self conceptions that include the "actual self," (attributes the individual actually possesses), "ideal self" (attributes the individual would like to possess), "ought self" (characteristics that someone else believes the individual should possess), and the "working self" (tentative self-conceptions tied to current circumstances). The working self-concept can be instantly accessed by the individual.

Possible Selves

Possible selves represent individuals' ideas of who they might become, who they would like to become, and who they are afraid of becoming. Possible selves provide organization, meaning, and direction to hopes, fears, goals, and threats (Markus & Nurius, 1986). Possible selves are drawn from past self representations and function as incentives for future behavior. They provide an evaluative and interpretive context for the self in the present. Individuals ardently avoid changing their self-concept. Thus possible selves may provide a conceptual link between cognition and motivation by providing a framework for change.

Positive possible selves are liberating because they provide hope that the present self can change. But negative possible selves are just as powerful because they can block attempts to change or develop. On the other hand, negative self-conceptions may be critical in initiating the process of self-concept change (Markus & Nurius, 1986). Possible selves serve as internal resources providing alternatives and options that allow individuals to temporarily ward off threats to self-esteem. Possible selves are differentially activated by the social situation and determine the nature of the working self-concept, contributing to the fluidity of the self (Marcus & Nurius, 1986).

The working self-concept is the basis for actions and observation, judgment, and the evaluation of intrapersonal and interpersonal actions. Intrapersonal actions include self-relevant information processing, affect regulation, and motivation. Interpersonal actions include social perception, social comparison, and interaction. "Variation in the content of an individual's working self-concept can have powerful consequences for mood, for temporary self-esteem, for immediately occurring thoughts and actions, and perhaps for more gradual long-term changes in self" (Marcus & Nurius, 1986, p. 964).

A discrepancy between who the self is and who it wants to be can motivate behavior (Markus & Wurf, 1987). In order to change behavior individuals must be able to self-regulate. Self-regulation includes those feelings (affective components) that influence goal selection, cognitive preparation for action, and behavior. Affective components are composed of diffuse innate needs, experiences, and self-conceptions; conscious values, and emotionally chosen behaviors; and specific learned motives, which drive unconscious and spontaneous behavior. Specific motives may include self-enhancement, developing or maintaining positive feelings about the self; self-consistency, providing coherence and continuity, or for self-actualization resulting in personal growth and development.

A shift in identity has been found to be a turning point in health behavior change (Kearney & O'Sullivan, 2003). A qualitative synthesis determined that a critical reevaluation of the self and the situation were vital to changing and sustaining behavior for 6 months or more. Initially, a growing body of evidence indicated that the impetus for a behavior change resulted from behavior outcomes incongruent with important values and goals. The health behavior itself was often not the source of distress, but rather distress resulted from the effects of the behavior on valued aspects of life (Kearney &

O'Sullivan, 2003). It was found that when small steps to change behavior were successful, more change followed through monitoring, judgment, and self-evaluation. This then strengthened the new identity and enabled new behaviors.

Schema Model of the Self-Concept

The schema model proposes that individual responses to stimuli are mediated through an internal system of content-specific organizations of knowledge (schemas) that are stored in long-term memory (Stein, 1995). Together, they form the individual's total collection of thoughts about the self. Schemas are derived from experience and reflect the way an individual constructs an event or object. Schemas are the foundation of purposeful thought and action, and are the organizing framework that gives meaning, form, and direction to an event. Self-schemas integrate and summarize an individual's thoughts, feelings, and experiences about the self in a specific behavioral domain. "Self-schemas are considered active, working structures that shape perceptions, memories, emotional, and behavioral responses" (Stein, 1995, p. 188). It can be hypothesized that self-schemas play a role in determining what information is noticed, how it is interpreted, and ultimately, which intervention is chosen.

Self-schemas are involved in action-planning, strategy selection, behavior rehearsal, knowledge repertoire, and automatic scripts. When a particular self-concept is activated, it is assumed that other closely related self-concepts will also be triggered. This increases the likelihood that the initial self-concept will be reactivated in the future (Marcus & Nurius, 1986). The process of internalizing content into a self-schema may be viewed as a continuum of incorporating content. This process begins with introjection, which moves the content inside the individual's mind but not into the self. Next, identification occurs, which begins the assimilation of the content into the self, and then integration makes the assimilation more complete (Carver & Scheier, 2000).

Self-schemas help individuals to process information about themselves in a particular sphere of influence. They also help the individual make decisions, and respond with behavior that is consistent with previous experience (Seigley, 1999). The influence of self-schemas on emotional and behavioral responses in specific domains has been supported by empirical evidence. Some models view self-schemas as static structures with definite boundaries and inner divisions (e.g., Shavelson), while others (e.g., Jung) view the "structure" as dynamic interrelationships or constellations (Jones, 2004). Self-schemas are somewhat fluid in nature, with new information creating changes in beliefs about the self. However, some aspects may be so important to the self that they are difficult or impossible to modify.

Self-schemas are an important means to bring about change. They help individuals to expand an unacknowledged strength and diminish the significance of vulnerabilities (Stein, 1995).

Bonham-Cheney Model of Self-Concept

The Bohman-Cheney self-concept model uses a systems approach. The concept of self is viewed as an open system composed of two interrelated subsystems, personal identity and self-perspective. These subsystems are divided into various components. Personal identity is made up of the *intellectual* self (all cognitive and creative functions), the *physical* self (structure, function, and appearance of the body), the *moral/ethical* self (personal belief and value systems), and the *emotional* self (feelings and attitudes). Self-perspective includes self-image (how I see myself), self-esteem (how I value myself), and self-in-action (how I use myself to interact with the environment). The two subsystems and their components comprise the self-concept and interact to affect the whole system. The system can change and adapt through feedback and through transfer of energy to balance negative threats with positive forces (Bonham & Cheney, 1983).

Status Dynamic Approach to Self-Concept

The "individual's self-concept is conceived as that individual's summary formulation of his or her status" (Bergner & Holmes, 2000, p. 36). The status dynamic view maintains that the self-concept is most usefully identified as a summary formulation, which is the individual's overall conception of their place in the scheme of things. This is in contrast to understanding the self-concept as an organized summary of perceived facts about the self. In the status dynamic approach, change is fundamentally about helping clients change the limiting, self-assigned categories that are often the source of their problems, and encouraging them to choose new categories with far more potential for behavior change.

Schema Assessment

Schema assessment is a framework that is primarily subjective, and reflects the client's (not the nurse's) perspective. This framework includes evaluating strengths as well as problems. Possible questions nurses can use with clients during a schema assessment include the following (Bonham & Cheney, 1983):

1. Are expectations unrealistic?
2. Are thoughts aligned with cognitive distortions? (e.g., I can't do well on this test.)
3. Are there objective data to support these thoughts? (e.g., I have studied for the test for days, but I still don't understand the material.)
4. Are "shoulds," "oughts," and "musts" being used to support maladaptive behavior? (Davidhizar & Shearer, 1996, p. 120). (e.g., I am exhausted, but I "must" stay up all night studying for the test.)

Implications for nursing intervention include some of the following considerations (Markus & Wurf, 1987):

1. Understand that clients tend to resist information that contrasts with their self-concept.
2. Enhance and promote the client's self-concept whenever possible.
3. Prefer and seek out positive information about clients.
4. Selectively interpret information to minimize a possible perceived threat by the client.
5. Help clients consider a positive view about the future.
6. Know that clients may adopt self-defeating actions that provide an excuse for failure.

7. Be aware that clients have selective attention, selective memory, and selective interpretation.
8. Understand that it is unclear when and how client self-representations will control behavior.
9. Help clients create specific positive options in the areas of concern. "Motivation can be viewed not as a generalized disposition or a set of task-specific goals, but as an individualized set of possible selves" (Marcus & Nurius, 1986, p. 966).

Self-Esteem

Self-esteem "is the affective component of the self" (Seigley, 1999, p. 74). Self-esteem results from an evaluation of how satisfied individuals are with their overall self-concept, reflecting the difference between how they would like to be (the ideal self) and how they actually are (the actual self) (King, 1997). Self-esteem is related to personal beliefs about skills, abilities, social relationships, and future outcomes. As individuals contemplate and evaluate themselves, self-esteem is experienced as an emotional response.

Girls are influenced by relationships (getting along), whereas boys are influenced by objective success (getting ahead). Women are more concerned than are men with body image (Heatherton & Wyland, 2003). An individual's self-esteem is stable because it slowly builds over time through personal experiences, but there can be fluctuations around a stable baseline.

Self-esteem can be affected by an overall evaluation or an assessment of specific aspects of the self. Aspects of the self that are often reviewed are *performance,* which includes general competence, self-confidence, efficacy, and sufficient agency to make the individual feel smart and capable; *social* skills are related to self-esteem and include how individuals believe they are perceived and how they interest and communicate effectively with others; *physical* attractiveness, which encompasses body image, race and ethnicity, and athletic skills; and a *summated* assessment of whether the individual feels good about the things that matter.

Outer self-esteem affects "temporary feelings of self-regard that vary over situations, roles, feedback, events, and the reflected appraisals of others" (Campbell, 1990, p. 539). In contrast, inner, or trait self-esteem is a global evaluation, a personal judgment of worthiness that appears to form relatively early in the course of development, remains fairly constant over time, and is resistant to change. Trait self-esteem is affected by positive and negative affective states; specific self-views, such as conceptions of strengths and weaknesses; and the relative certainty and importance of self-views strongly linked to personally important goals and values (Pelham & Swann, 1989).

Two antecedents to self-esteem include how the individual perceives the appraisal of significant others, and feelings of competence, which are derived from how effectively the individual can affect the environment (Seigley, 1999). Self-esteem can be evaluated by the ability to influence significant others; receiving acceptance and affection from significant others; successfully performing to meet the demands of significant others; and adherence to moral and ethical standards communicated through the environment (Seigley, 1999). Leary and MacDonald (2003) describe several labels associated with self-esteem, including:

1. *State self-esteem*—the way individuals feel about themselves at a particular moment in time.
2. *Trait self-esteem*—how individuals most typically feel about themselves.
3. *Global self-esteem*—how individuals feel about themselves overall.
4. *Collective self-esteem*—the social identity individuals gain from belonging to certain groups.
5. *Implicit self-esteem*—an individual's potentially biased capacity to accurately report their attitudes and feelings.

MULTICULTURAL COMPETENCY

In modern Western societies, identity is personally and individually constructed, so that the individual can be distinguished from others. This identity must be continually verified, reexamined, updated, and defended. In more homogeneous, traditional, or Eastern cultures, identity is more closely linked to an individual's age, gender, status, caste, or roles, and is embedded in relationships. The individual's negotiated place in a social network is the main form of reality (Cross & Gore, 2003).

A cultural frame refers to an interpretive schema, grid, or meaning system. It consists of language and a set of tacit social understandings or norms that are the understandings of daily social representations and practices (Marcus & Kitayama, 1994). Social behavior that is consistent with a given cultural norm eventually comes to feel "good" (Markus & Kitayama, 1994). Cross and Gore (2003) discuss the following cultural norms for behavior in social networks. These networks have a major influence on individual self-esteem and confidence.

1. The assumption that autonomy and personal choice are the major contributors to high levels of motivation applies primarily to individuals from Western backgrounds. Asian Americans prefer choices made by a close and valued in-group.
2. In Japan, socially skilled individuals avoid directly expressing choices and opinions and they sidestep choices when they are offered (enryo).
3. East Asians are much more tolerant of inconsistency, ambiguity, and contradiction. Their culture values a balance of contradictory forces that can be reconciled through compromise.
4. Euro-Europeans tend to seek direct or primary control over their environments, whereas East Asians tend to try to adjust to their environments and to display indirect or secondary control.
5. In East Asian cultural contexts, the primary standard for evaluating the self is how well the individual meets the cultural norms of fitting into important groups, behaving appropriately in social situations, and maintaining harmony in relationships.

Several specific cultural norms are discussed here. For example, in Chinese, two terms approximate some of the meanings associated with self-esteem. One is "zi zun xin" in Mandarin or "chu chun sim" in Taiwanese, which can be literally translated into English as "self-respect-heart/mind." The second related term is "zi xin xin" in Mandarin or "chu sin sim" in Taiwanese, the literal English translation of which is "self-confidence-heart/mind" (Miller, Wang, Sandel, and Cho, 2002, p. 228).

Among African Americans, social support and self-reliance are the two predominant and interconnected self-esteem needs. Social support comes from families, friends, churches, and communities. Other self-esteem–related themes include pride, respect, a positive outlook, and the use of self-talk (DeFrancisco & Chatham-Carpenter, 2000). Self-talk seems consistent with and is encouraged by traditional African oral cultures. For African Americans the concept of self is fundamentally community based.

Elements of a sense of identity and self-esteem in African American females, developed through both individual and collective accomplishments, are a sense of control, especially as it relates to dealing with racism, and a sense of belonging or interdependence (DeFrancisco & Chatham-Carpenter, 2000). "African American girls tend to have higher self-esteem than do Caucasian and Hispanic American girls…African American women do not tend to internalize negative body images to the degree that Caucasian women do" (DeFrancisco & Chatham-Carpenter, 2000, p. 74). The unifying philosophic concept in the African American experience is the notion of family unity, connectedness, and inter-dependence. Belonging to a group, cooperation, and collective responsibility are the norm rather than individuality, competitiveness, and independence. Central to the family are faith and church.

American females (except for African American females) have been found to have lower levels of both global and public domain self-esteem than males. Yet, self-esteem is much more important in American mothers' folk theories of childrearing than it is in their Taiwanese counterparts. "For Taiwanese mothers, self-esteem is either not something that mothers worry very much about, or it is believed to create psychological vulnerabilities rather than strengths" (Miller et al., 2002, p. 209). Taiwanese mothers do not seem to cultivate the child's individuality for its own sake. Either individual differences are accepted as a matter of course, or moral guidance is individualized.

INTERVENTIONS

Listed below are some illogical and distorted ideas about self-esteem that may affect a client's thinking. Understanding these distortions enables the nurse to help clients evaluate and adjust their thinking. Illogical and distorted ideas can include:

1. Perceiving circumstances only in black-and-white categories
2. Exaggerating or minimizing events, situations, or personal qualities
3. Over-generalizing or basing behavior on a single negative event or situation
4. Participating in selective negativism or being preoccupied with an issue or event that blots out any productive logical thinking
5. Making assumptions or attempting mind-reading or fortune-telling without objective data to support conclusions
6. Negating positive thought, rejecting positive experiences, and maintaining negative beliefs
7. Reasoning with emotions, resulting in decisions and self-evaluation based on negative thinking (Davidhizar & Shearer, 1996)

It has been proposed that convincing individuals of the importance of their positive self-views should be an especially effective method of raising low self-esteem (Pelham & Swann, 1989).

Not having enough data to evaluate a situation accurately is very distressing and may lower self-confidence (Davidhizar & Shearer, 1996). Self-talk may be used as a way to restructure thinking, but infrequent self-talk is usually not effective. Reframing or shifting illogical labeling can be used by the nurse to move clients toward problem-solving and a positive use of countering techniques. These techniques are aimed at challenging the client's thinking or changing negative thought patterns to foster increased self-confidence. For example, countering techniques could include:

- Decreasing distress by visualizing a pleasant scene or using relaxation techniques
- Using thought-stopping techniques, such as clapping hands or snapping a rubber band at the wrist
- Becoming neutral by getting rid of distractions, distorted thoughts, and preoccupations
- Visualizing a positive outcome
- Mental rehearsal of positive thoughts (positive self-talk) (Davidhizar & Shearer, 1996).

Other helpful strategies that promote positive thinking and enhance confidence include listening for recurrent negative themes and changing them, modeling positive thinking, and reading books and attending workshops. Recognizing the beginning signs of positive thinking and giving the self more positive feedback also will help to reinforce positive thoughts and feelings (Davidhizar & Shearer, 1996, p. 122).

References

Bergner, R. M., & Holmes, J. R. (2000). Self-concepts and self-concept change: A status dynamic approach. *Psychotherapy: Theory, research, practice, training, 37*, 36–44.

Bonham, P. A., & Cheney, A.M. (1983). Concept of self: A framework for nursing assessment. In P. L. Chinn (Ed.), *Advances in nursing theory development* (pp. 173–190). Rockville, MD: Aspen.

Campbell, J. D. (1990). Self-esteem and clarity of the self-concept. *Journal of Personality and Social Psychology, 59*, 538–549.

Carver, C. S., & Scheier, M. F. (2000). Autonomy and self-regulation. *Psychological Inquiry, 11*, 284–291.

Cross, S. E., & Gore, J. S. (2003). Cultural models of the self. In M. R. Leary & J. P. Tangney (Eds.), *Handbook of self and identity* (pp. 536–564). New York: Guilford Press.

Davidhizar, R. E., & Shearer, R. (1996). Increasing self-confidence through self-talk. *Home Healthcare Nurse, 14*, 119–122.

DeFrancisco, V. L., & Chatham-Carpenter, A. (2000). Self in community: African American women's views of self-esteem. *The Howard Journal of Communications, 11*, 75–92.

Hanton, S., Meilalieu, S. D., & Hall, R. (2004). Self-confidence and anxiety interpretation: A qualitative investigation. *Psychology of Sport and Exercise, 5*, 477–495.

Heatherton, T. F., & Wyland, C. L. (2003). Assessing self-esteem. In S. J. Lopez, & C. A. Snyder (Eds.), *Positive psychological assessment: A handbook of models and methods* (pp. 219–233). Washington DC: American Psychological Association.

Jones, R. (2004). The science and meaning of the self. *Journal of Analytical Psychology, 49*, 217–233.

Kear, M. (2000). Concept analysis of self-efficacy. Retrieved 5/5/04, from http://www.graduatere search.com/Kear.htm.

Kearney, M. H., & O'Sullivan, J. (2003). Identity shifts as turning points in health behavior change. *Western Journal of Nursing Research, 25,* 134–152.

King, K. A. (1997). Self-concept and self-esteem: A clarification of terms. *The Journal of School Health, 67,* 68–70.

Leary, M. R., & MacDonald, G. (2003). Individual differences in self-esteem: A review and theoretical integration. In G. MacDonald, M. R. Leary, & J. P. Tangney (Eds.), *Handbook of self and identity* (pp. 401–418). New York: Guilford Press.

Markus, H., & Nurius, P. (1986). Possible selves. *American Psychologist, 41,* 954–969.

Markus, H., & Wurf, E. (1987). The dynamic self-concept: A social psychological perspective. *Annual Review of Psychology, 38,* 299–337.

Markus, H. R., & Kitayama, S. (1994). The cultural construction of self and emotion: Implications for social behavior. In S. Kitayama & H. R. Markus (Eds.), *Emotion and culture: Empirical studies of mutual influence* (pp. 89–130). Washington DC: American Psychological Association.

Miller, P. J., Wang, S., Sandel, T., & Cho, G. E. (2002). Self-esteem as folk theory: A comparison of European American and Taiwanese mother's beliefs. *Parenting: Science and practice, 2,* 209–239.

Pelham, B. W., & Swann, W. B. Jr. (1989). From self-conceptions to self-worth: On the sources and structure of global self-esteem. *Journal of Personality and Social Psychology, 57,* 672–680.

Roy, C. (1987). Roy's adaptation model. In R. R. Parse (Ed.), *Nursing science: Major paradigms, theories, and critiques* (pp. 35–45). Philadelphia: WB Saunders.

Seigley, L. A. (1999). Self-esteem and health behavior: Theoretic and empirical links. *Nursing Outlook, 47,* 74–77.

Stein, K. F. (1995). Schema model of the self-concept. *Image: Journal of Nursing Scholarship, 27,* 187–193.

CHAPTER 11

Power Part Six: Capacity

Concepts
Capacity
Unitary Energy
Vital Energy
Metabolic Energy

Figures & Tables
Table 11-1 Noninvasive Therapies

Models and Theories
Leddy's Energetic Patterning Nursing
    Practice Theory

Interventions
Thought Field Therapy

Helpful Lists
Mutual Process Energetic Patterning,
    pgs. 133–134
Components of Thought Field Therapy,
    pg. 136

Thought Questions
1. What is the difference between vital and metabolic energy? What are their purposes?
2. What is a "field of energy"? How do the nurses' field and the clients' field influence each other?
3. Describe the "anatomy" of the vital energy field. What are the purposes of meridians, chakras, and nadis(s)?
4. Discuss the domains of the energetic nursing practice theory. Which noninvasive nursing interventions fit with each domain?
5. How can the nurse assist client self-healing through both the vital and metabolic energy fields?

Chapter Synopsis
This chapter introduces the concept of capacity as a human strength and as a resource for health. Capacity is closely related to the Healthiness Theory concepts of goals, choice, capability, and control. Two fields of energy, the vital field and the metabolic field are described. Leddy's Nursing Theory of Energetic Patterning is discussed, and the intervention of thought field therapy is outlined. In addition, many of the noninvasive therapeutic modalities proposed in the theory of energetic patterning are relevant to facilitating movement and harmony of the energy fields.

Sections of this chapter were previously published (2003) in *Visions: The Journal of Rogerian Scholarship, 11,* 21–28. They are reprinted with permission of the editor.

A UNITARY PERSPECTIVE OF ENERGY

Capacity is composed of both vital and metabolic energy (discussed later). The concepts of a unitary perspective of energy were discussed in Chapter 2. These concepts include (a) universal essence, which is composed of particle and wave, and interchangeable facets: *matter,* which is the potential for structure and identity; *information,* which is the potential for coordination and pattern; and both vital and metabolic *energy,* which are potentials for process, movement, and change; (b) field, which is a nonobservable domain of influence; pattern; oscillation of waves that determine frequency, amplitude, and resonance of energy; and synchronization and conscious focusing of energy vibrations. It has been proposed that the nurse can facilitate health patterning by fostering resonance of environmental (vital) energy and information (Leddy, 2003a).

It is proposed here that universal essence is manifested in two energy fields, vital energy and metabolic energy. *Vital energy,* is associated with the informational aspect of universal essence, and ensures the individual's cohesiveness and unity. *Metabolic energy* is associated with the matter aspect of universal essence and includes the processes that ensure the effective functioning of the individual. Capacity, as it is conceptualized in this book, requires the integration of vital and metabolic energy, although the ways in which these energy fields engage in mutual processes have yet to be articulated.

Capacity energizes a "quantity" of material matter and initiates the movement necessary for process. Capacity is an active strength that is expressed in vigor and vitality. Peterson and Seligman (2004, p. 273) describe vitality as "a dynamic aspect of well-being marked by the subjective experience of energy and aliveness." Capacity can be decreased by factors such as conflict, stress, illness symptoms (e.g., pain and fatigue), and poor nutrition. It can be increased by contact with outdoor and natural environments, relatedness, enjoyable physical activity, a nutritious diet, and noninvasive therapeutic modalities (e.g., meditation, yoga, and imagery) that enhance calmness and harmony.

Capacity has a reciprocal relationship with goals, choice, capability, and control strengths in the Healthiness Theory. Capacity "energizes" the other strengths, just as it is rejuvenated by them.

The Structure of the Vital Energy Field

A detailed picture of the human universal essence field has been described by Gerber (1988) and Kunz and Peper (1982), where the individual is conceptualized as a series of interpenetrating, interactive, and multidimensional fields. These fields include the physical body, viewed as a "complex energetic interference pattern of interwoven energy fields" (Gerber, 1988, p. 60). According to Gerber (1988) within the physical body, and intertwined in the same space are fields of increasingly subtle, higher energetic frequencies. It has been suggested that "through thoughts and intention, the…field can be stretched to considerable distances, such as ten to fifteen feet...Relaxation tends to expand the field while anxiety tends to constrict the field" (Kunz & Peper, 1982, p. 400). Energy constantly circulates within the body in 12 well-defined channels, or physical ducts called meridians, which exist as a series of points following line-like patterns. Energy always moves from high to low potential from more to less energy (Gerber, 1988). The meridian system is believed to facilitate energy and information interconnections throughout the human field.

Special energy centers known as *chakras* exist within the human universal essence field. Chakras (Sanskrit meaning wheels), "resemble whirling vortices of subtle energies, that 'take in' higher energies and transmute them to a utilizable form within the human structure" (Gerber, 1988, p. 128). There are at least seven major chakras associated with the physical body, in a vertical line ascending from the base of the spine to the head. These are the root chakra (I) near the coccyx, the sacral chakra (II) located either just below the umbilicus or near the spleen, the solar plexus chakra (III) in the upper middle abdomen below the tip of the sternum, the heart chakra (IV) in the midsternal region directly over the heart and the thymus, the throat chakra (V) directly over the thyroid gland and larynx, the brow chakra (VI) in the region of the mid-forehead slightly above the bridge of the nose, and the crown chakra (VII) located on the top of the head. Each is associated with a major nerve plexus and a major endocrine gland (Gerber, 1988).

Because chakras separate vibrations into various frequencies, a specific color, tone, function, organ, and nervous structure has been associated with each chakra. Chakras seem to be responsible for receiving, processing, transforming, and transmitting energy and information that may be stored in the higher frequency fields (Slater, 1995).

Connecting the chakras to each other and to portions of the physical-cellular structure are up to 72,000 fine subtle-energetic channels, known as *nadis*. These are interwoven with the physical nervous system (Gerber, 1988). "Nadis, or channels of electromagnetic energy, subdivide finally to the cellular level, supporting the concept that healing can affect the cellular level of the physical body" (Starn, 1998, pp. 211–212). All of the cells in the body are linked together in what has been called a "living matrix" (Oschman, 2000). The meridian/chakra/nadis system channels energy to the cellular level where the energy is transformed to support specific biochemical cellular functions, and also changed into information that is communicated throughout the individual. "The living matrix has no fundamental unit or central aspect, no part that is primary or most basic. The properties of the whole net depend upon the integrated activities of all the components" (Oschman, 2000, p. 48).

An Energy–Based Nursing Practice Theory

The Energetic Patterning Nursing Practice Theory (Leddy, 2003b) proposes that healing nursing interventions assist field energy movement and resonant patterning of both the client and the nurse healer. Six domains of the mutual process energetic patterning (participation) underlying healing nursing interventions have been identified:

1. *Connecting*—fosters harmony with the environmental field and within the human field.
2. *Coursing*—clears meridians to reestablish free movement of energy.
3. *Conveying*—fosters redirection of energy away from areas of excess to depleted areas.

4. *Converting*—amplifies resonance to augment resources.
5. *Conserving*—decreases disorder or flux to reduce areas of energy depletion.
6. *Clearing*—transforms matter to release energy tied to old patterns (Leddy, 2003a).

A number of interventions are consistent with this theory. Selected noninvasive interventions for each domain of participation are listed in Table 11-1.

Energy healing occurs in the human essence field, which is the physical body. When field patterns are disrupted by blockage, deficiency, or excess, illness is manifested in the body. "All diseases are caused by a break in the flow or a disturbance in the human energy field" (Hunt, 1996, p. 77), manifesting in the field long before becoming obvious in the body (Starn, 1998). The American Nursing Diagnosis Association (NANDA), classified "energy field disturbance" as a legitimate nursing diagnosis. However, by defining it as "a disruption of the flow of energy *surrounding* a person's being which results in disharmony of the body, mind, and/or spirit" (emphasis added) the NANDA has not understood

Table 11-1. **Noninvasive Therapies**

CLEARING	COURSING
Music/color therapy	Massage
Acupressure	Yoga
Postural movement	Polarity Therapy
Aromatherapy	Exercise
CONVEYING	**CONVERTING**
Acupressure	Nutrition
Reflexology	Herbal Therapy
	Music/color therapy
	Exercise
CONSERVING	**CONNECTING**
Relaxation/meditation	Guided imagery
Biofeedback	Reiki
Sleep and rest	Therapeutic Touch
Breathing	Aromatherapy
Herbal therapy	Music/color therapy

1. *Connecting.* Promotes harmony of energetic patterning.
2. *Coursing.* Reestablishes free movement of energy.
3. *Conveying.* Fosters redirection of energy away from excess to depleted areas.
4. *Converting.* Transforms and augments energy resources.
5. *Conserving.* Reduces energy depletion.
6. *Clearing.* Releases energy tied to old patterns.

Source: Leddy, S. K. (2003). *Integrative health promotion: Conceptual bases for nursing practice.* Thorofare, NJ: Slack Inc.

Rogers' (1980) admonition that individuals do not *have* energy fields, they *are* energy fields (emphasis in the original).

Healing is based on a view of human-environment process as mutual and open. Actual physical touch and "exchange" of energy are not needed for energetic healing because of the integrality of the human-environment essence fields of the client and the practitioner. The field process may be experienced as a cool breeze, a tingling or prickling feeling, a pulsation, a vibration, heat, or other changes in temperature, an expanding force, electricity (sensation of light static), pressure, or magnetism. It is often not necessary for the healer to "do" anything. The client is able to self-heal through resonance with appropriate energy frequencies. In other words, the client's field incorporates energy frequencies that enhance self-healing with the healer acting as a facilitator or booster to accelerate the client's healing process (Sharp, 1997).

Leddy (2003b) theorizes that intentional focus by the healer can foster harmonious entrainment of energy field vibration. "Attention may increase synchronization of bio-physical processes, creating a laser-like summation of energy" (Schwartz & Russek, 1997, p. 54). The actual mechanism for energy healing may be a bioelectronic wave that moves between healer and client, initiated by intention or expectation in the nurse healer (Leddy, 2003a). "The healer with a strong field, focused through intent, will provide a coherent powerful energy field" (Hunt, 1996, p. 269). Or, the healer may focus human/environment field energy by placing their hands very near, not necessarily touching the physical body of the person being treated. "What we do is assist individuals to transform or change their unique energy form and in so doing, purposively actualize inherent potentials" (Todaro-Franceschi, 1999, p. 2). By providing a range of appropriate energy frequencies, and "entraining the oscillations back to coherence" (Oschman, 2000, p. 135) field balance and harmony often can be restored. Universal essence field harmony is associated with healthiness and healing.

Elements of the Metabolic Energy Field

Metabolic energy is derived from protein, carbohydrate, and fat food sources through both anabolic and catabolic processes. These food sources are irregular, so they need to be regulated by the brain, pancreas, liver, skeletal muscle, and adipose tissue. These sites provide ways to store energy at times of surplus, and provide energy at times of need. ATP (adenosine triphosphate) serves as the energy source at the cellular level. Each cell must continuously synthesize its own ATP to meet its energy needs. ATP is synthesized from the breakdown of glycogen and fat (Copstead & Banasik, 2000).

The key to regulation of blood levels of glucose is appropriate insulin secretion from pancreatic B-cells, effective suppression of lipid mobilization and utilization, and activation of diverse metabolic pathways of tissue energy uptake and storage (Storlien, Oakes, and Kelley, 2004). Skeletal muscle, adipose tissue, and the nervous and endocrine systems play major roles in energy balance and flexibility. Hormones that affect metabolism of glucose include insulin, glucagon, growth hormone, glucocorticoid hormones (epinephrine and norepinephrine), and thyroid hormone.

Three physiological systems interact to promote cell-cell communication: the nervous, endocrine, and immune systems. For example, the nervous system plays an important role in regulating the synthesis and secretion of a variety of hormones within specific endocrine systems. Cytokines are synthesized and released by specific immune and non-immune cells, and play an important role in the regulation of a variety of immunological as well as neuroendocrine processes (Demas, 2004). Energy balance and immune function are linked, as immune responses require energy. Consequently, reductions in energy availability suppress immunity.

Adipose tissue serves as an important endocrine organ. Reductions in total body fat are correlated with impaired immunity, and seasonal changes in immune function correlate with seasonal fluctuations in total body fat (Demas, 2004). In addition, leptin acts as a neuroendocrine signal, communicating current energy availability, whether in the form of readily utilizable energy (i.e., glucose) or energy stores. An important role of the sympathetic nervous system is to regulate the effects of leptin on immune function (Demas, 2004, p. 173).

The capacity for self-regulation appears to be limited. Self-control also depends on a limited resource, akin to energy or strength. For example, willpower contributes to a strength or energy reserve. Acts of self-control and, more generally, of choice and volition, deplete this resource and impair the self's ability to function (Baumeister, 2002). Resources that are expended by acts of self-control and volition are gradually replenished, primarily through sleep and rest. Positive emotions also seem to have some value for replenishing the self's stock of energy and its capacity for self-regulation (Baumeister, 2002).

INTERVENTIONS

Thought Field Therapy

"Perturbations can be experienced energetically as disruption along an energy meridian" (Gallo, 2002, p. 6). Callahan has developed an intervention to promote coherent, dynamic resonance between and among meridians, known as Thought Field Therapy. The components of thought field therapy are:

1. *Muscle testing and therapy localization* (applied kinesiology).
2. *Thought field attunement* (psychological reversal of polarity)—consists of affirmation statements while tapping or touching acupoints.
3. *Tapping at acupuncture sites* (meridian acupoints); or touch and breathe—consists of light touch with one to four fingers on a specific acupoint while taking one breath through the nose.
4. *Nine-gamut treatments*—consists of touch or tapping on the gamut spot on the back of the hand under nine conditions: eyes closed and eyes open, eyes down and to the right and eyes down and to the left, rotating the eyes 360 degrees first clockwise and then counterclockwise, humming a tune for a few seconds, counting aloud from one to five and then humming again. This procedure stimulates different areas of the brain.
5. *Eye roll treatment*—consists of scanning with the eyes from top to bottom while tapping on the gamut spot on the back of the hand.
6. *Collarbone breathing procedure*—consists of a specific breathing pattern with activation of specific meridians (Gallo, 2002).

References

Baumeister, R. F. (2002). Ego depletion and self-control failure: An energy model of the self's executive function. *Self and Identity, 1,* 129–136.

Copstead, L. C., & Banasik, J. L. (2000). *Pathophysiology: Biological and behavioral perspectives* (2nd ed.). Philadelphia: WB Saunders.

Demas, G. E. (2004). The energetics of immunity: A neuroendocrine link between energy balance and immune function. *Hormones and behavior, 45,* 173–180.

Gallo, F. P. (2002). *Energy psychology in psychotherapy.* New York: W. W. Norton & Company.

Gerber, R. (1988). *Vibrational medicine.* Santa Fe, NM: Bear & Co.

Hunt, V. V. (1996). *Infinite mind: Science of the human vibrations of consciousness.* Malibu, CA: Malibu Publishing.

Kunz, D., & Peper, E. (1982, December). Fields and their clinical implications. *American Theosophist, 70,* 395–401.

Leddy, S. K. (2003a). *Integrative health promotion: Conceptual bases for nursing practice.* Thorofare, NJ: Slack Inc.

Leddy, S. K. (2003b). A nursing practice theory: Applying a unitary perspective of energy. *Visions: The Journal of Rogerian Scholarship, 11,* 21–28.

Oschman, J. L. (2000). *Energy medicine: The scientific basis.* Edinburgh: Churchill Livingstone.

Peterson, C., & Seligman, M. E. P. (2004). Vitality. *Character strengths and virtues: A handbook and classification* (pp. 273–289). Washington, DC: American Psychological Association.

Rogers, M. E. (1980). Nursing: A science of unitary man. In J. P. Riehl & C. Roy (Eds.), *Conceptual models for nursing practice* (2nd ed., pp. 329–331). New York: Appleton-Century-Crofts.

Schwartz, G. E., & Russek, L. G. (1997). Dynamical energy systems and modern physics: Fostering the science and spirit of complementary and alternative medicine. *Alternative Therapies, 3,* 46–56.

Sharp, M. B. (1997). Polarity, reflexology, and touch for health. In C. M. Davis (Ed.), *Complementary therapies in rehabilitation* (pp. 235–255). Thorofare, NJ: Slack Inc.

Slater, V. E. (1995). Toward an understanding of energetic healing, Part 2: Energetic processes. *Journal of Holistic Nursing, 13,* 225–238.

Starn, J. R. (1998). The path to becoming an energy healer. *Nurse Practitioner Forum, 9,* 209–216.

Storlien, L., Oakes, N. D., & Kelley, D. E. (2004). Metabolic flexibility. *Proceedings of the Nutrition Society, 63,* 363–368.

Todaro-Franceschi, V. (1999). *The enigma of energy: Where science and religion converge* (p. 2). New York: Crossroad Publishing.

CHAPTER 12

Health Strengths Outcomes

Concepts
Well-Being
Hardiness
Quality of Life

Models and Theories
Ryff's Model of Psychological Well-
  Being
Oishi's Goal Approach to Well-
  Being
Marcus and Kitayama's Model
  of Well-Being
Process Theory
Kovac's Quality of Life Model
Health-Related Quality of Life

Systems Control Analysis Approach
Social Support

Interventions
Well-Being Therapy
Cultural Considerations of Quality
  of Life

Helpful Lists
Characteristics of Cultural Syndromes,
  pgs. 144–145
Helping Clients to Change Thoughts
  and Beliefs, pgs. 145–146
Socio-Psychological Agents of Quality
  of Life, pg. 148

Thought Questions
1. How do well-being, satisfaction, happiness, and quality of life differ?
2. What are the differences between languishing, flourishing, and floundering
   patterns of well-being manifestations? What are the implications for nursing
   practice?
3. What are the dimensions of Ryff's Model of Psychological Well-Being? Describe
   at least one implication for nursing practice for each dimension.
4. How does culture affect perceptions of well-being and quality of life?
5. What domains of quality of life do you think are important for nursing interventions? How can the environment specifically affect quality of life?

Chapter Synopsis
This chapter introduces the concepts of well-being and quality of life as outcomes when
human strengths are used as resources for health. Multiple human strength theories, such
as Ryff's model of psychological well-being, Oishi's goal approach to well-being, process
theory, social production functions theory, social support, Kovac's quality of life model,

and health-related quality of life are described. Aspects of multicultural competency are mentioned. Finally, limitations of existing intervention strategies and issues for clarification of the quality-of-life concept are discussed.

WELL-BEING

Subjective well-being (SWB) is based on an affective and cognitive evaluation of an individual's life. The perception of health is influenced by subjective well-being, which consists of positive affect, negative affect, and life satisfaction (Diener, Lucas, and Oishi, 2002; Lightsey, 1996). The components of subjective well-being have been identified as life satisfaction (i.e., global judgments about life), satisfaction with important domains (e.g., work satisfaction), positive affect (i.e., experiencing many pleasant emotions and moods), and low levels of negative affect (i.e., experiencing few unpleasant emotions and moods) (Diener, 2000; Schalock & Alonso, 2002). "Although SWB is not sufficient for the good life, it appears to be increasingly necessary for it" (Diener, 2000, p. 34). SWB and its correlates show striking gender similarities across cultures (Lightsey, 1996).

Subjective well-being is related to the common but often vaguely defined term "happiness." However, Ryff (1989) questions the emphasis on the hedonistic feeling of "happiness." She suggests an alternative definition of SWB as those feelings consistent with true potential, a sense of an excellence, or a perfection toward which the individual strives. According to Ryff (1989) components of well-being include self-acceptance; intimacy, and generativity, denoting positive relationships with others; autonomy demonstrated by an internal locus of control; environmental mastery; a clear comprehension of life's purpose, a sense of direction, and intentionality that contributes to purpose in life; and an openness to experience and personal growth.

Well-being and happiness are sometimes considered interchangeable concepts. An individual's long-term happiness level is governed by three kinds of factors: a fixed happiness set point that is difficult but not impossible to change; happiness-relevant circumstances, such as location, income, and marital status; and intentional, cognitive, motivational, and behavioral strategies that are feasible but difficult to implement (Lyubomirsky & Abbe, 2003). Happiness includes a sense that life is good, meaningful, and worthwhile combined with an experience of joy, contentment, or positive well-being (Lyubomirsky, 2001).

Happiness and satisfaction are closely related and both are embedded in the research on subjective well-being. Happiness represents one component of satisfaction, and reflects affect associated with positive and negative emotions and moods. Satisfaction represents global judgments about life, including such subdomains as work or health. Satisfaction demonstrates a trait-like stability over time, in contrast with happiness which tends to be more transitory (Schalock & Alonso, 2002).

It is not clear whether it is possible to reinforce or enhance an individual's personal happiness or if sustainable increases in happiness are even attainable. But it is known that positive emotions increase the likelihood of feeling good in the future, and that individuals who feel good live longer (Fredrickson, 2003). It has been found that even unrealistically optimistic beliefs are associated with greater longevity, whereas beliefs reflecting the realistic acceptance of the likelihood of death are associated with a faster course of disease (Lyubomirsky & Abbe, 2003).

Research has shown that "physicians experiencing positive emotion tend to make more accurate diagnoses; that optimistic people are more likely than pessimists to benefit from adverse medical information; that in presidential elections over the past century, 85% were won by the more optimistic candidate; that wealth is only weakly related to happiness, both within and across nations; that trying to maximize happiness leads to unhappiness; that resilience is experienced by many people; and that nuns who display positive emotions in their autobiographical sketches live longer and are healthier over the next 70 years" (Seligman & Pawelski, 2003, p. 162).

Well-being can be described as patterns of languishing, flourishing, or floundering (Keyes & Lopez, 2002). Languishing is a low level of well-being. In contrast, individuals who are flourishing have high levels of emotional, psychological, and social well-being. Individuals with mental disorders are described as floundering in life because they have an illness and generally very low levels of emotional, psychological, and social well-being. However, many individuals who have an illness may also be filled with moderate or high levels of emotional, psychological, and social well-being, which is described as a state of struggling with life (Keyes & Lopez, 2002). This view of well-being has been called eudemonia, which is defined as "the feelings accompanying behavior in the direction of and consistent with, one's true potential...an ideal in the sense of excellence, a perfection toward which one strives, and it gives meaning and direction to one's life" (Ryff, 1989, p. 1070).

High income, individualism, feeling that human rights are valued, and social equality are connected with the sense of well-being. On the cultural level the SWB is associated with attributes of entities such as gross national income per capita, average longevity, and percentage of national income spent on the environment. The personal level refers to the individual's attitudes, beliefs, perceptions, and values. Individuals react strongly to good and bad events, but over time they adapt and then return to their original level of happiness (Diener, 2000). Environmental mastery and autonomy increase from young adulthood to old age. Purpose in life and personal growth decrease from young adulthood to old age. Self-acceptance and positive relationships with others show little age variation.

Predictors of subjective well-being include a combination of personal characteristics and social-cultural factors, such as extroversion, meeting intellectual challenges, social belonging and social support, health, religiosity, personal freedom, and being reasonably affluent. But in most countries, the correlation between income and happiness is negligible.

Temperament and personality appear to powerfully influence an individual's sense of well-being. Lasting happiness may come, in part, from activities such as working for personal goals (see Chapter 4), participating in close social relationships (see Chapter 5), experiencing physical and mental pleasures, and being involved in "flow" (see Chapter 9) activities. Contrary to popular belief, making more money seems to contribute little to the sense of well-being.

RELATED CONCEPTS

Hardiness

The concept of hardiness is a summation of the concepts of commitment, challenge, and control. "Empirical evidence does not support hardiness theory" (Lightsey, 1996, p. 631).

THEORIES

Ryff's Model of Psychological Well-Being

Ryff (1989) suggests that psychological functioning should be assessed in terms of concepts she believes to be universal: self-acceptance, personal growth, purpose in life, positive relations with others, environmental mastery, and autonomy. The individual who scores high in *self-acceptance* possesses a positive attitude toward the self; acknowledges and accepts multiple self aspects including good and bad qualities; and feels positive about the past. The individual who scores low in self-acceptance feels dissatisfied with the self; is disappointed with the past; is troubled about certain personal qualities; and wishes to be different.

The individual with a high score in *positive relations* with others has warm, satisfying, trusting relationships; is concerned about the welfare of others; is capable of strong empathy, affection, and intimacy; and understands the give and take of relationships. In contrast, the individual with a low score has few close trusting relationships; finds it difficult to be warm, open, and concerned about others; is isolated and frustrated in interpersonal relationships; and is not willing to compromise to sustain important personal ties.

The individual with a high score in *autonomy* is self-determining and independent; is able to resist social pressures to think and act in certain ways; regulates behavior from within; and evaluates the self based on personal standards. The individual with a low score is concerned about the expectations and evaluations of others; relies on judgments of others to make important decisions; and conforms to social pressures to think and act in certain ways.

The individual with a high score in *environmental mastery* has a sense of mastery and competence in managing the environment; controls a complex array of external activities; makes effective use of surrounding opportunities; and is able to choose or create contexts suitable to personal needs and values. The individual with a low score has difficulty managing everyday affairs; feels unable to change or improve the surrounding context; is unaware of opportunities; and lacks a sense of control over the external world.

The individual who scores high in *purpose in life* has goals in life and a sense of direction; finds life meaningful in both the past and present; and has beliefs that give life purpose. The individual with a low score lacks a sense of meaning in life; has few goals or aims; lacks a sense of direction; does not see purpose in the past; and has no outlook or beliefs that give life meaning.

And finally, the individual who scores high in *personal growth* has a feeling of continued development; sees the self as growing and expanding; is open to new experiences; has a sense of realizing personal potential; sees behavior improve over time; and is changing in ways that reflect greater self-knowledge and effectiveness. The individual who scores low has a sense of personal stagnation; lacks a sense of improvement or expansion over time; feels bored and uninterested with life; and feels unable to develop new attitudes or behaviors (Ryff, 1989, p. 1072).

Oishi's Goal Approach to Well-Being

Goal researchers take into account individual differences and developmental shifts in markers of well-being. Values, which are guiding principles in life, are considered higher order goals. Lower order goals include personal strivings, which are defined as the activities done in daily life. Oishi (2000) assumes that markers of well-being (e.g., autonomy) vary across individuals, depending on their goals and values.

A study by Oishi (2000) found cultural differences in the attributes of well-being. These findings raise some questions about the universality of the self-determination theory and Ryff's model of well-being. Descriptors of well-functioning individuals show systematic cultural variation. This indicates that different cultures and social environments have different modes of behaviors, values, and attitudes that are suited for adjustment in particular societies. Thus, social contextual theories of well-being need to be developed that are based on a clear understanding of the role of culture in shaping an individual's sense of well-being.

Marcus and Kitayama Model of Well-Being

The Marcus and Kitayama model of well-being (Marcus & Kitayama, 1994), based on cultural psychology, maintains that the nature of "good feelings" differs from culture to culture, depending on each culture's view of the self. For example, in Japan, it was found that good feelings typically resulted from meeting obligations and expectations and involved friendliness and feeling fulfilled. But in the United States, good feelings typically involved pride and satisfaction from achieving personal goals. This suggests that "the degree to which individuals engage in normative behaviors determines their life satisfaction" (Oishi, 2000, p. 104).

Both the Marcus and Kitayama model and Oishi's goal approach predict cultural variations in the determination of the sense of well-being. But there are important differences in each model's approach to the role of culture. Marcus and Kitayama suggest that culture prescribes acceptable behaviors, and when the individual follows the prescribed behavior they feel satisfied. This model does not suggest much variation between individuals within the same culture. On the other hand, the goal as moderator model suggests that culture influences the type of goals individuals pursue, and that individuals are satisfied with life to the extent that they are moving toward their goals. The goal as moderator model also allows for individual differences in the sources of well-being within a culture (Flores & Obasi, 2003).

Unfortunately, available data do not allow a direct test of the difference between these models. Across nations there are differences in total population ratings of subjective well-being (see following). Individualistic-oriented cultures scored higher than collectivistic cultures, and wealthier nations scored higher than poorer nations.

Process Theory

Process Theory (Lightsey, 1996) uses the term *process* to convey the idea of an individual as a dynamic system that exists only in relation to the environment. Making a personal or environmental appraisal entails using the rational processing system. This processing system is governed largely by the cerebral cortex, which includes conscious thoughts and beliefs, and the experiential processing system, which includes schemata. Schemata are content-specific organizations of knowledge stored in long-term memory that are an individual's total collection of cognitions about the self. Particular appraisals of the environment always lead to particular emotions that are specific to the appraisals. Schemata are strongly tied to emotion, however, behavior also regulates and may directly promote emotion. Preexisting positive (goal-striving) or negative (harm-avoidance) feelings activate schemata and moderate the effect of subsequent stressors on the immune system or health. Process theory provides a unified framework that accounts for many findings and places personal resources in the larger context of human functioning.

MULTICULTURAL COMPETENCY

Evaluating whether a society is successful depends on what criteria are used when making the assessment. Different societies have different sets of values, and each society will use the criteria relevant to that society. The concept of cultural relativism thus points to the need for internal standards when judging societies. This leads to questions about whether citizens of a society are able to accomplish goals consistent with their values, and if they can use their own standards to judge whether their lives and communities are successful (Diener & Suh, 1999).

Individuals in individualistic nations naturally consult their feelings when deciding how satisfied they are, and feeling pleasant emotions frequently is a reasonable predictor of life satisfaction in these societies. In collectivist cultures individuals tend to evaluate their lives based on norms that set standards for satisfaction and consider the social appraisals of family and friends (Diener, 2000). Some countries are better able to meet the basic needs for food, clean water, and health. Culture also influences the individual's goals and values. Finally, culture affects optimism and positive feelings, social support, coping patterns, and the degree of regulation of personal desires.

Cultural Syndromes

"A cultural syndrome is a shared pattern of attitudes, beliefs, categorizations, self-definitions, norms, role definitions, values, and other subjective elements of culture that is organized around some theme" (Triandis, 2000, p. 29). Those who speak a particular language or dialect, live during a particular historic period, or who reside in a definable geographic region might exhibit a cultural syndrome. Characteristics of cultural syndromes include:

1. *Complexity/simplicity*— affects the number of roles and choices available.
2. *Tightness/looseness*—affects sanctions or tolerance for deviating from norms; tightness is expected to be associated with a lower sense of well-being.
3. *Individualism/collectivism*— affects how central the individual is in the culture.

Individualism is associated with a higher sense of well-being, high self-esteem and optimism. "People in collectivist cultures are extremely supportive of their in-group members, but they have cold, and even hostile, relationships with out-group members...They arrange things so as to make it difficult for strangers to develop interpersonal trust" (Triandis, 2000, p. 29).

Forces that increase sense of well-being at the cultural level include: high gross national product per capita; political freedoms; social equality; social security; satisfactory citizen-bureaucrat relationships; high levels of trust; and efficient public institutions. Forces that increase sense of well-being at the individual level include: good health; sufficient education; a fit between personality and culture; a personality open to new experiences; extroversion; conscientiousness; environmental mastery; personal growth; purpose in life; self-acceptance; sense of self-determination; opportunities to compare the self favorably to others; having many acquaintances; receiving social support from many close friends; and less stress (Triandis, 2000).

According to an economic approach, well-being will be greater in a nation with higher productivity (more goods, services, and fulfillment of human needs) (Diener & Suh, 1999). Gross domestic product per capita of 55 nations and the level of the sense of well-being have a moderate correlation (Diener & Suh, 1999). Individualism also has a high correlation with national wealth. These findings beg the question why? Does satisfaction with material goods influence other aspects of life, or do wealthy nations have other characteristics (e.g., equality) that directly lead to satisfaction?

Some nations express a greater sense of well-being more than others. On a scale of 1 to 10, with 10 the highest, Bulgaria scored 5.03; Russia scored 5.37; Denmark scored 8.16; Switzerland 8.39; and U.S. scored 7.71, all near the top in SWB. But are nations a meaningful level of analysis? There are indications that the influences of nationality remain stable so that the sense of well-being appears to be homogenous within a nation. The sense of well-being seems to vary with a balance between the individual's orientation toward the self and toward others, interpersonal trust, and political stability. "A widespread feeling of well-being is necessary for democracy to prosper" (Diener & Suh, 1999, p. 448).

Despite some variation, the sense of well-being is high in all countries (Triandis, 2000). In developed countries the correlation between the sense of well-being and self-esteem is high, whereas in the less developed countries it is low. "It may be that when basic needs are satisfied, self-esteem is salient, but when basic needs are not satisfied, self-esteem is not salient, so it does not correlate with SWB" (Triandis, 2000, p. 17). In China and India, suffering is seen as part of being human, it can be ennobling and is associated with good feelings. The relevant cultural frame influences normative coping practices and desirable feeling states, and therefore is a necessary factor in research on the sense of well-being (Markus & Kitayama, 1994).

INTERVENTIONS

Well-Being Therapy

Well-being therapy is a short-term, well-being enhancing psychotherapeutic strategy. Therapy goals are not necessarily the reduction of symptoms but increased personal comfort and effectiveness (Fave, 1999). The strategy extends over eight sessions, and takes place weekly or every other week. The duration of each session ranges from 30 to 50 minutes. The technique emphasizes self-observation, through the use of a structured diary, and interaction between the client and nurse. It is structured, directive, problem-oriented, and based on an educational model. Techniques include cognitive restructuring (modification of automatic or irrational thoughts); scheduling of activities (mastery, pleasure, and graded task assignments); assertiveness training; and problem-solving.

The initial sessions are concerned with identifying and placing episodes of well-being into a situational context. The client uses the diary to write down the circumstances surrounding episodes of well-being, recording each event regardless of its length. In the intermediate sessions, the client is encouraged to identify thoughts and beliefs leading to a premature interruption of well-being (e.g., I have so much to do). At this point, the nurse can challenge these thoughts with appropriate questions, such as what is the evidence for or against an idea. Or, the nurse might choose to reinforce and encourage activities likely to elicit well-being in the client. The intent of this therapy is for the client to be self-monitoring. The nurse should refrain from suggesting conceptual and technical alternatives. In the final sessions, errors in thinking and alternative interpretations are discussed, using Ryff's framework.

Changing Thoughts and Beliefs

Counseling must achieve its effects first via changes in positive and negative thoughts and beliefs about the self and outcomes (Lightsey, 1996). Suggestions for nurses to use when helping clients change thoughts and beliefs include:

1. Concentrate on helping clients to develop self efficacy (being able to influence their own thoughts and behavior) and goals at specific and general levels. The ultimate goal should be to help clients to change schemata to include more self-efficacious beliefs.
2. Use a variety of interventions to increase efficacy beliefs, through graded mastery experiences, verbal persuasion, vicarious learning, and having the client interpret their physiological/emotional state.
3. Use verbal persuasion early in counseling.
4. Integrate homework that uses graded but powerful mastery experiences in domains valued by the client (e.g., finish homework for school, or pay all bills).
5. Encourage the client's expression of positive and negative emotions. Increased emotional disclosure is associated with decreased sympathetic activity and increased immune system activity.
6. Help the client to increase positive thoughts/beliefs and to decrease negative thoughts/beliefs. Strive for a preponderance of positive thinking relative to negative thinking.
7. Help the client to develop active problem-solving skills.
8. Teach a variety of coping skills.
9. Use a variety of modalities to effect change in schemata, including information, persuasion, and confidence-building. Use visual imagery that is closely tied to stimulation of schemata.
10. Cultivate knowledge of the client's culture.

11. Do not lose sight of human commonalities across cultures.
12. As a nurse/counselor pay attention to personal emotions and find an outlet for their expression.

Self management strategies include self-monitoring, self-instruction, self-evaluation, self-reinforcement, goal-setting and attainment, problem-solving, and observational learning.

QUALITY OF LIFE

Quality of life (QOL) concerns well-being in a broad sense (Gerritsen, Steverink, Ooms, and Ribbe, 2004). However, QOL has been described as "a patchwork of dimensions with poor theoretical connections between them" (Dupuis, Taillefer, Etienne, Fontaine, Boivin, and Von Turk, 2000, p. 254) and thus tends to have a diffuse meaning. Many terms such as happiness, satisfaction, performance, functioning, goal-attainment, needs satisfaction, health, and well-being are used to designate QOL.

Quality of life is composed of the same factors and relationships for all individuals. Individuals experience QOL when their needs are met and when they have opportunities to pursue life enrichment in major life settings. Although, QOL has both subjective and objective components, it is primarily reflected by the individual's feelings about his or her quality of life.

Quality of life is a multidimensional concept, based on individual needs, choices, and control, and influenced by individual and environmental or contextual factors (Schalock & Alonso, 2002). Definitions of QOL frequently include emotional well-being, health, intimacy issues, and work and activities related to productivity. It has been suggested that QOL life indicators may have to be weighted by the subjective valuing and importance to the life domain (Wrosch & Scheier, 2003).

Through using their abilities or achieving a productive lifestyle, individuals can satisfy their values, goals, and needs. Both quality of life and successful development might be supported through pursing attainable goals and disengaging from unattainable goals (Wrosch & Scheier, 2003). Lawton defined QOL in frail, elderly people as "the multidimensional evaluation, by both intra-personal and social-normative criteria, of the person-environment system of an individual in time past, current, and anticipated" (Lawton, 1991, p. 6). In other words, QOL includes both personal and social criteria and is time dependent. He distinguished four independent sectors of QOL, *behavioral* competence (competent functioning in the health, cognitive, time-use, and social dimensions); *domain-specific* perceived QOL (subjective evaluation of function in the behavioral competence dimensions); *objective* environment (physical and intrapersonal); *psychological* well-being "the weighted [by the self] evaluated level of the person's competence and perceived quality in all domains of contemporary life" (Lawton, 1991, p. 11).

There are several models or paradigms of QOL, including the *scientific* or biomedical paradigm where curing the disease process is the focus; the *functional* model, which emphasizes rehabilitating the individual for maximum functioning; and the *environmental* model in which interacting with the environment affects personal limitations. There is a social responsibility to eliminate systemic social, economic, and physical barriers that affect an individual's participation in the civil and social rights of a society. Social responsibility can include advocating for and providing political and social entitlements to enhance the well-being and quality of life for those on the fringes of society.

The World Health Organization Project (WHOQOL, 1997), used a medical model when it assumed that the QOL is formed from six domains: physical health; psychological health; level of independence; social relationships; environment; and spirituality/religion/personal. Through an extensive review of the literature, Schalock (2004) identified eight core QOL domains: emotional well-being; interpersonal relations; material well-being; financial status; personal development; physical well-being; self-determination; social inclusion; and rights.

However, Dupuis and colleagues (2000, p. 251) insist that quality of life must be defined without reference to domains. "Dimensions [domains] are accessories, epiphenomena [secondary phenomenon]…The focus on dimensions has led the field to a dead end." They suggest that QOL should be defined without reference to domains, with the resulting operational definition later applied to domains.

Societal/Environmental (Ecological) Perspective

The societal-level application of the QOL concept is multifaceted. It is a complex interaction among individuals, programs, and public policies implemented at the societal level to enhance the well-being of individuals. Decreased functional ability "is neither fixed nor dichotomized; rather it is fluid, continuous, and changing within an evolving set of personal characteristics that depend on the services and supports available to the person" (Schalock & Alonso, 2002, p. 334). Intervention, services and/or supports should focus on adaptive behavior, role or community status, and subjective well-being.

The German ecological-environmental lexicon (Katalyse, 1993) lists 15 areas that determine or affect health and thereby the QOL predominantly in civilized countries. These include agriculture; air; chemicals; dwelling; earth; energy; free-time; industry; health; noise; radiation; transportation; waste; wood; and work.

The Dutch sociologist Veenhoven (2000) analyzed nine areas of socio-psychological agents of quality of life. These are:

1. *Material wealth*—buying power compared with other countries
2. *Living standard*—especially nutrition, safe drinking water, etc.
3. *Protection of individuals*—incidence of suicides, fatal accidents, corruption, violence, and vandalism
4. *Freedom*—political freedom and respecting of civil rights
5. *Social equality*—gender and discrimination of minorities
6. *Cultural climate*—percentage of individuals striving for higher education, access to information, value orientation, and cultural and spiritual life
7. *Social climate*—tolerance toward others, trust toward institutions, individuals in positions of authority, social participation, and armament costs
8. *Population pressure*—increasing population density, especially in the cities
9. *Modernization*—urbanization, industrialization, and emphasis on information transmission

   The National Program Office on Self-Determination at the University of New Hampshire designed an environmental initiative to enhance quality of life by restructuring the long-term care system in the United States. This initiative proposed moving from a facility-based, highly regulated system to individualized funding arrangements where individuals and their advocates have control over money and services. Four principles of self-determination are being implemented by this agency: (a) freedom for individuals to choose where and with whom to live and how to spend their time, (b) authority to control the money and budget needed for support while the money moves with the individual, (c) support that is organized according to the individual's specific needs and desires, and (d) responsibility for the wise use of public funding and for contributing to the community (Schalock & Alonso, 2002).

The Environmental Context

Environmental factors can help individuals realize their full potential, accomplish positive life goals, and achieve an enduring sense of well-being (Stokols, 2003). Some of the physical and social environments that can positively affect well-being include places that evoke pleasurable experiences, environments that are easy to navigate and do not cause confusion or disorientation, and beautiful or tranquil natural settings. Environments that can negatively affect well-being include noisy, overcrowded and heavily trafficked settings; a lack of privacy; social isolation; and natural and technological disasters. The duration of the exposure to the environment obviously affects either its positive or negative impact.

   Environmentally based enhancement techniques especially for the disabled include user-friendly environments that meet the environmental needs of individuals. For examples, wheelchair-accessible sidewalks and buildings; signs with Braille in public buildings; opportunities for community involvement; easy access to outdoor environments; modifications to stairs, water taps, doorknobs; safety measures (e.g., handrails, safety glass, nonslip walking surfaces); convenience measures (e.g., orientation aids such as color coding or universal pictographs); accessibility to a home and the community; sensory stimulation (e.g., windows, less formal furniture); prosthetics (e.g., personal computers, specialized assistance devices); and opportunities for choice and control (e.g., lights, temperature, privacy and personal space). Additional examples include: building codes, principles of barrier-free design, adapted curricula, and policy and funding commitments targeted to remove or resolve specific barriers (Schalock & Alonso, 2002).

THEORIES

Kovac's Quality of Life Model

Kovac's QOL model (Kovac, 2003) has three levels, a basal (existential—all human) level, mezzo (individually specific—civilization) level, and a meta (elite—cultural/spiritual) level. The basal level consists of at least six areas of life including a normal physical state, normal mental functioning, a functional family, material/social security, a life-giving environment, and the basic skills necessary for survival. Each part of the basal level of QOL has its qualitatively higher representation at the mezzo- and/or meta-levels.

However, the model does not specify the relationships between individual components of the quality of life. The meaning of life is created by an integration of cognitive, emotional, and motivational components. "The discovered and developed meaning of life is such a prime regulator of individual components of QOL that it is also the most effective source of man's permanent satisfaction with life, a source of continuous well-being, a forum where moments of happiness can appear for brief periods of time" (Kovac, 2003, p. 95). Kovac believes that religiosity, a personal positive approach to God and transcendence, is at the core of meaning of life. Religiosity, or spirituality, involves cognition (religious beliefs), experiencing (religious feelings), and action (religious rituals and cults).

Social Production Functions Theory

According to the social production functions (SPF) theory (Lindenberg, 1986), individuals will strive for well-being, despite constraints, by achieving universal and specific goals. Goals are hierarchical, with each level instrumental to the level above. "QOL (or psychological well-being) is the ultimate and overall goal for an individual and is the result of the realization of [both] physical and social well-being [universal goals]" (Gerritsen et al., 2004, p. 618). In the first level below the universal goals there are five first-order instrumental goals: *stimulation* (a pleasant amount of stimulation and activation); *comfort* (the satisfaction of basic physical needs and the absence of health complaints, safety concerns, and fear); *affection* (being loved); *behavioral confirmation* (doing the right things); and *status* (being appreciated). As the individual ages, it is predicted that status is probably the first goal that is discarded, then stimulation and behavioral confirmation. When the last remaining resources for comfort and affection become threatened, QOL is seriously endangered.

Health-Related Quality of Life

Schalock and Alonso (2002) describe three levels of health-related quality of life (HRQOL): *personal* (subjective level of satisfaction); *functional* (objective interaction with a neighborhood, community, or organization); and *social* (external, environmentally based, i.e., health, social welfare, standard of living, education, public safety, housing, neighborhood, leisure). They propose that the levels include physical well-being (physical status and symptoms, autonomy, physical capacity); psychological well-being; functional (occupational) ability; general health perception and well-being; and social activity. They also suggest end motives for QOL, such as independence (desire for self-reliance); power (desire for influence, mastery, leadership, and dominance); honor (desire to be loyal to parents, ethnic group, or heritage); order (desire for a predictable environment); status (desire for social standing); acceptance (desire to be included); social contact (desire for interaction with others); tranquility (desire to be free of anxiety, fear, or pain); curiosity (the desire to explore or learn); exercise (the desire for physical movement); and saving (the desire to collect) (Schalock and Alonso, 2002).

Social Support and Quality of Life

Structural measures of the environment deal with the existence of social relationships (e.g., marital status, number of friends, frequency of interaction with friends, number of roles an individual has). *Functional* measures refer to the resources provided by others within an individual's social network, such as emotional support (having others available to listen, care, sympathize, and who provide reassurance, value, and love); *instrumental* support (assistance, such as help with household chores, lending money, or running errands); or *informational* support (information or guidance) (Helgeson, 2003).

The stress-buffering hypothesis states that the relation of social support to QOL depends upon the individual's level of stress. If there is no stress or little stress, social support is unrelated to QOL. Under conditions of high stress, however, social support serves as a buffer against the adverse effects of stressors. It is believed that emotional support is the strongest stress buffer, especially for uncontrollable stress.

There are three phases in the timing of a stressor. During each of these phases the nurse can play an active role in supporting clients. In the crisis phase, the client becomes aware of a stressor as being threatening; this is when emotional support may be most needed. During the transitional phase, the client actually copes with the stressor, and requires information. In the deficit phase, the client is overwhelmed and may need instrumental support. Perceived support is more strongly related to QOL than received support. Social relationships can also be a source of conflict, stress, and tension (support burdens, unintended support failures).

INTERVENTIONS

It is unclear whether the cognitive and motivational processes associated with relatively greater happiness can be nurtured, acquired, or directly taught. This is a significant question because heritability coefficients as high as 50% to 80% have been identified for happiness, whereas objective circumstances, demographic variables, and life events only account for 8% to 15% of the variance in happiness (Lyubomirsky, 2001). Happy individuals use different cognitive, judgmental, and motivational strategies than those who are unhappy.

Consequently, several factors need to be determined including: the identification of effective and enduring ways to retrain cognitive and motivational strategies; how to maintain successful gains and, perhaps, even to initiate an upward spiral; and how to enhance happiness without forfeiting goodness or truth (Lyubomirsky, 2001). At this time there is little evidence for the effectiveness of using peer discussion group interventions to enhance happiness.

Cultural Considerations of Quality of Life

The following questions might form a structure to consider a future agenda for clarification of the QOL concept:

1. What is the relative importance of each core QOL domain and core indicator within different countries and cultures?
2. What is the degree to which each domain and core indicator is either used by service providers or experienced by service recipients?
3. Why does the QOL concept "play out" better in some countries than in others? Is it an issue of the "haves" and "have nots;" of collectivism versus independence; or

a different emphasis on autonomy and individual liberty versus liberty, fraternity, or equality?

4. What are the cultural adaptations of the QOL concept? Which cultural factors facilitate the application of the QOL concept, and which factor(s) inhibit or preclude its cultural acceptance and inclusion?

References

Diener, E. (2000). Subjective well-being: The science of happiness and a proposal for a national index. *American Psychologist, 55,* 34–43.

Diener, E., Lucas, R. E., & Oishi (2002). Subjective well-being. In C. R. Snyder, & S. J. Lopez (Eds.), *Handbook of positive psychology* (pp. 63–73). Oxford: Oxford University Press.

Diener, E., & Suh, E.M. (1999). National differences in subjective well-being. In D. Kahneman, E. Diener, & N. Schwartz (Eds.), *Well-being: The foundations of hedonic psychology* (pp. 434–450). New York: Russell Sage Foundation.

Diener, E., & Suh, E. M. (2000). *Culture and subjective well-being.* Cambridge, MA: MIT Press.

Dupuis, G., Taillefer, M. C., Etienne, A. M., Fontaine, O., Boivin, S., & VonTurk, A. (2000). Measurement of quality of life in cardiac rehabilitation. In J. Jobin, F. Maltais, P. LeBlanc, & C. Simard (Eds.), *Advances in cardiopulmonary rehabilitation* (pp. 247–273). Champaign, IL: Human Kinetics.

Fave, G. A. (1999). Well-being therapy: Conceptual and technical issues. *Psychotherapy and Psychosomatics, 68,* 171–179.

Flores, L. Y., & Obasi, E. M. (2003). Positive psychological assessment in an increasingly diverse world. In S. J. Lopez & C. R. Snyder (Eds.), *Positive psychological assessment: A handbook of models and measures* (pp. 41–54). Washington, DC: American Psychological Association.

Fredrickson, B. L. (2003). The value of positive emotions. *American Scientist, 91,* 330–335.

Gerritsen, D. L., Steverink, N., Ooms, M. E., & Ribbe, M. W. (2004). Finding a useful conceptual basis for enhancing the quality of life of nursing home residents. *Quality of Life Research, 12,* 611–624.

Helgeson, V. S. (2003). Social support and quality of life. *Quality of Life Research, 12,* (Suppl. 1), 25–31.

Katalyse, E. V. (1993). *Umweitlexikon, Instit fur angewandte:* Umweiltforschung, Koln.

Keyes, C. L. M., & Lopez, S. J. (2002). Toward a science of mental health. In C. R. Snyder & S. J. Lopez (Eds.), *Handbook of positive psychology* (pp. 45–59). Oxford: Oxford University Press.

Kovac, D. (2003). Quality of life: A paradigmatic challenge to psychologists. *Studia Psychologica, 45,* 81–101.

Lawton, M. P. (1991). A multidimensional view of quality of life in frail elders. In J. E. Birren, J. E. Lubben, J. C. Rowe, & D. E. Deutchman (Eds.), *The concept and measurement of quality of life in frail elders* (pp. 3–27). San Diego, CA: Academic Press.

Lightsey, O. R. (1996). What leads to wellness? The role of psychological resources in well-being. *The Counseling Psychologist, 24,* 589–735.

Lindenberg, S. (1986). The paradox of privatization in consumption. In A. Diekman & P. Mitter (Eds.), *Paradoxical effects of social behavior* (pp. 297–310). Heidelberg/Vienna: Physica-Verlag.

Lyubomirsky, S. (2001). Why are some people happier than others? The role of cognitive and motivational processes in well-being. *American Psychologist, 56,* 239–249.

Lyubomirsky, S., & Abbe, A. (2003). Positive psychology's legs. *Psychological Inquiry, 14,* 132–136.

Markus, H. R., & Kitayama, S. (1994). The cultural construction of self and emotion: Implications for social behavior. In S. Kitayama & H. R. Markus (Eds.), *Emotion and culture: Empirical studies of mutual influence* (pp. 89–130). Washington DC: American Psychological Association.

Oishi, S. (2000). Goals as cornerstones of subjective well-being: Linking individuals and cultures. In E. Diener & E. M. Suh (Eds.), *Culture and subjective well-being* (pp. 87–112). Cambridge, MA: MIT Press.

Ryff, C. D. (1989). Happiness is everything, or is it? Exploration on the meaning of psychological well-being. *Journal of Personality and Social Psychology, 57,* 1069–1081.

Schalock, R. L. (2004). The concept of quality of life: What we know and do not know. *Journal of Intellectual Disability Research, 48*(Part 3), 203–216.

Schalock, R. L., & Alonso, M. A. V. (2002*). Handbook on quality of life for human service practitioners.* Washington DC: American Association on Mental Retardation.

Seligman, M. E. P., & Pawelski, J. O. (2003). Positive psychology: FAQs. *Psychological Inquiry, 14,* 159–163.

Stokols, D. (2003). The ecology of human strengths. In L. G. Aspinwall & U. M. Staudinger (Eds.), *A psychology of human strengths: Fundamental questions and future directions for a positive psychology* (pp. 331–343). Washington DC: American Psychological Association.

Triandis, H. C. (2000). Cultural syndromes and subjective well-being. In E. Diener, & E. M. Suh (Eds.), *Culture and subjective well-being* (pp. 13–36). Cambridge, MA: MIT Press.

Veenhoven, R. (2000). Freedom and happiness: A comparative study in forty-four nations in the early 1990s. In E. Diener & E. M. Suh (Eds.), *Culture and subjective well-being* (pp. 257–288). Cambridge, MA: MIT Press.

WHOQOL. (1997). *Measuring quality of life.* Geneva: World Health Organization.

Wrosch, C., & Scheier, M. F. (2003). Personality and quality of life: The importance of optimism and goal adjustment. *Quality of Life Research, 12*(Suppl. 1), 59–72.

CHAPTER 13

Health Behavior Change Theories

Concepts
Stages and Processes of Change
Decisional Balance
Self-Efficacy
Locus of Control
Health Beliefs

Figures & Tables
Figure 13-1 Health Behavior Change Model
Table 13-1 Main Concepts of the Prominent Theories of Health Behavior (Change)
Table 13-2 Titles, Definitions, and Representative Interventions of the Processes of Change

Models and Theories
Transtheoretical Model
Health Behavior Change Model
Health Behavior Goal Model
Modified Health Belief Model
Revised Health Promotion Model
Self-Efficacy Theory
Theory of Reasoned Action
Theory of Planned Behavior
Theory of Locus of Control
Common Sense Model
Behavioral Initiation/Maintenance Stage Theory
Pender's Health Promotion Model

Helpful Lists
Assumptions of the Transtheoretical Model, pgs. 160–161
Six Stages of Behavior Change, pgs. 161–162
Steps in the Change Process, pg. 162
Stages of Change and Interventions, pg. 165
Influences on Self-Efficacy, pgs. 166–167
Health Beliefs, pg. 168
Health Promotion Model Influences, pg. 169

Thought Questions
1. What concepts are used across the various models and theories? What is the evidence to support the usefulness of these concepts?
2. What are the stages of change?
3. Describe at least one process that is appropriate for each stage of change.
4. How can self-efficacy and internal locus of control be used to promote individual behavior change?
5. How can health beliefs influence stages of behavior change?

Chapter Synopsis
This is the first of two chapters dealing with individual behavior change. This chapter addresses multiple concepts and theories that attempt to explain behavior change (or its lack) in individuals. The theories discussed include stages and processes of the Transtheoretical model, the Behavioral Initiation/Maintenance Stage Theory, Decisional Balance, Self-Efficacy, Locus of Control, Health Beliefs, the Health Promotion Model, and The Health Behavior Goal Model. This content is followed by implementation strategies to promote individual behavior change in Chapter 14.

Portions of this chapter, reprinted with the permission of the publisher, have previously been published in Leddy, S. K. (2003) *Integrative Health Promotion: Conceptual Bases for Nursing Practice.* Thorofare, NJ: Slack Inc.

INDIVIDUAL BEHAVIOR CHANGE

It is not easy for individuals to change their lifestyle and adopt healthy behaviors. Current behaviors indicate negative health trends resulting in obesity, tobacco use, low physical activity, and poor diet (Orleans, 2000). For example, the prevalence of obesity in the United States rose from 25% of the population in the 1960s to about 33% in 2000 (Jeffery, Drewnowski, and Epstein, 2000). Physical activity begins declining at about age 6 and continues throughout life, with about 70% of adults over age 45 getting no regular exercise (Marcus et al., 2000). Only 25% of adult Americans meet the dietary goal of 30% or less of calories from fat, and sodium intake is increasing (Kumanyika et al., 2000). Another concern is that only about one-third of patients correctly follow physician directions (Clark & Becker, 1998).

Obviously if individuals are going to adopt healthy behaviors, more effective ways are needed to promote, support, and maintain changes in behavior. The following section describes a number of theories addressing the factors and strategies that influence behavior change.

THEORIES OF BEHAVIOR CHANGE

In order to encourage and support healthy behaviors, nurses need to understand how and why individuals change their behavior. A number of complex models use belief system and social cognitive theories to explain individual behavior change. Belief system theory views personality structure as an organization of beliefs, attitudes, and values about the self and others (Quackenbush, 2001). Cognitive theory, in contrast, argues that emotions and problems are primarily due to the individual's thought processes, whereas social cognitive theories assume that personal, social, and environmental influences interact to affect and change behavior. Prominent belief system and cognitive models and theories are listed in Table 13-1.

- *Transtheoretical Model* (Prochaska, & DiClemente, 1984)—proposes that stages and processes of change, decisional balance, and self-efficacy influence stopping an unhealthy behavior or adopting a healthy behavior.

Table 13-1. Main Concepts of the Prominent Theories of Health Behavior (Change)

	HEALTH BELIEF MODEL	ROTTER'S SOCIAL LEARNING THEORY	THEORY OF REASONED ACTION/ THEORY OF PLANNED BEHAVIOR (TPB)	BANDURA'S SOCIAL LEARNING THEORY	PROTECTION MOTIVATION THEORY
Personal characteristics	Demographic- and sociopsychological factors internal cues to action				
Environmental characteristics	External cues to actions	Situation/social context			
Threat appraisal	Health threat · Perceived susceptibility · Perceived severity				· Perceived susceptibility · Perceived severity
Perceived benefits	Perceived benefits of action	· Reinforcement (overall expectancy) · Reinforcement value	Attitude to behavior · Probability of (positive) outcome · Value of outcome	Outcome—expectancy	· Response—efficacy
Perceived costs	Perceived barriers to action		Attitude to behavior · Probability of (negative) outcome · Value of outcome		· Costs (or perceived barriers) · Internal rewards of current behavior · External rewards of current behavior

(continued on following page)

Table 13-1. Main Concepts of the Prominent Theories of Health Behavior (Change) *(Continued)*

	HEALTH BELIEF MODEL	ROTTER'S SOCIAL LEARNING THEORY	THEORY OF REASONED ACTION/ THEORY OF PLANNED BEHAVIOR (TPB)	BANDURA'S SOCIAL LEARNING THEORY	PROTECTION MOTIVATION THEORY
Social influence			Subjective norms · Normative beliefs · Motivation to comply		
Perceived competence		Locus of control	Perceived behavioral control (only in TPB) · Probability of control factor · Power of control factor	Self-efficacy	Self-efficacy
Mediating processes	Likelihood of taking health action	Behavior potential	Behavioral intention	Probability of behavior	Protection motivation

Source: From Moes, S., & Gebhardt, W. (2000). Self-regulation and health behavior: The health behavior goal model. In M. Boekaerts, P. R. Pintrich, & M. Zeidner (Eds.), *Handbook of self-regulation* (pp. 343–363). San Diego, CA: Academic Press. Used with permission of the Publisher.

- *Health Behavior Change Model* (Leddy, 2004)—describes motivators, mediators, and maintenance of behavior change by blending healthiness theory (Leddy, 1996) with the stages and processes of change and decisional balance concepts from the Transtheoretical model. This model is shown below in Figure 13-1.
- *Health Behavior Goal Model* (Boekaerts, Pintrich, and Zeidner, 2000)—integrates stages and values, such as health and emotional costs and benefits, social influence, personal and environmental sources of change, and perceived competence, with goal expectancies.
- *Modified Health Belief Model* (Rosenstock, Strecher, and Becker, 1988)—proposes that the perception of susceptibility and seriousness of the health threat affects the individual's perception of disease. This perception, combined with the possible benefits and barriers to action, affects the likelihood of a preventative health action being taken.
- *Revised Health Promotion Model* (Pender, 1996)—depicts individual characteristics, experiences, and behavior-specific thinking that affect and influence healthy behavior.
- *Self-Efficacy Theory* (Bandura, 1986)—is concerned with an individual's judgments about the ability to execute given levels of performance and to exercise control over events.
- *Theory of Reasoned Action* (Fishbein & Ajzen, 1975)—emphasizes the effects of attitude and subjective norms on behavioral intention and actual behavior.
- *Theory of Planned Behavior* (Ajzen, 1985)—adds perceived behavioral control to the effects of attitude and subjective norms on behavioral intention and actual behavior.
- *Theory of Locus of Control* (Rotter, 1954)—proposes that individuals either believe that their action controls an outcome (internals), or that they are controlled by forces other than themselves (externals), such as chance or powerful others.
- *Theory of Health Locus of Control* (Wallston, Maides, and Wallston, 1976)—proposes an inclination toward acting in health-related situations based on an individual's perception of having control over his or her health and the valuing of health as an end in itself or as a means to a different end.
- *Common Sense Model* (Leventhal, Meyer, and Nerenz, 1980)—proposes that common sense beliefs, about identity, causes, timelines, consequences, and cure or control of illness guide how individuals cope with health problems. These beliefs direct attention to information and serve as a basis for selecting coping strategies.

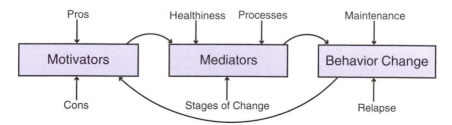

Figure 13-1. Health Behavior Change Model.

Criticism

Subjective utility models, such as the Health Belief Model, Theory of Reasoned Action, and Theory of Planned Behavior, which focus on the usefulness of behavior, are criticized for the following reasons:

- Not incorporating emotional processes
- Viewing behaviors as static events rather than dynamic processes that change over time
- Not delineating feedback processes for evaluating progress toward or away from goals

Criticisms of stage theories of health behavior, which view behavior change developmentally, include:

- Not delineating the roles of emotional processes in influencing behavior
- Not considering the nature of psychological processes within the stages
- Not considering the influence of the social and environmental context on behavior change
- Defining beliefs, attitudes, emotional experiences, and social factors as pros and cons. But by doing so, these theories obscure the complexities of cognitive, affective, and social processes (Cameron & Leventhal, 2002)

The scientific literature has viewed the various models and theories as competing. As a result, studies have compared the ability of concepts within a theory or model to explain or predict behavior change. The emphasis has been on determination of the "best" predictor theory or model. But it is now clear that there is a great deal of conceptual overlap among the various theories and models. In addition, it appears that a complex network of constructs may predict only a portion of each behavior and these networks vary from one behavior to the other. In most studies, much of human behavior is not explained (AbuSabha & Achterberg, 1997).

Another approach is to study the concepts that appear *across* models and theories, to understand how the influences on a specific behavior and across a variety of behaviors might be combined for a broader explanation. The following section will explore a number of hypotheses that have demonstrated potential to explain or predict behavior change.

STAGES OF CHANGE

The Transtheoretical Model

Stages and processes of change are two of the four concepts in the Transtheoretical Model (TTM). Stages of change (discussed following) reflect motivational, social learning, and behavior relapse theories. Six basic assumptions of this stage model are (Laitakari, 1998, p. 32):

1. Change in health behavior happens through distinct stages or steps.
2. Change takes place optimally in a certain order of stages.

3. Completing the previous stages promotes the reaching of the subsequent stages. For example, completion of the preparation stage is necessary before entering the action stage.
4. There are factors that promote adoption (e.g., "processes" or "supporting-factors") specific to each stage. These are discussed later in this chapter.
5. The stage-specific factors can be mobilized through intervention methods (e.g., "techniques") to speed up the process of adoption. These are discussed later in this chapter.
6. Relapse is possible after reaching a stage, but relapse can be used to provide valuable information to help the individual make a new attempt to change. For example, many individuals stop exercising after several weeks or months. But, understanding the reasons for "relapse" can be very helpful in revising the exercise plan to support success with the next effort.

A consistent series of six stages of behavior change (see following) have been documented across 12 different health-related behaviors (Prochaska, DiClemente, and Norcross, 1992; Prochaska, Velicer, et al., 1994). The same pattern of change among TTM variables across stages was documented in a cross-sectional study of high school and undergraduate university students and employed adults (Rodgers, Courneya, and Bayduza, 2001). Males and females differed in stage of change for exercise. Men were more likely than females to be in the maintenance stage (see definition later) of change for exercise, whereas females were more likely than males to be in the contemplation stage of change (see following). Males reported fewer cons for adopting regular exercise, but they also reported significantly fewer pros (O'Hea, Wood, and Brantley, 2003).

- *Precontemplation* is the stage where the individual has no intention of changing behavior in the next 6 months. Resistance to recognizing or modifying a problem is the hallmark of precontemplation. The optimal strategy for moving individuals from precontemplation to contemplation is to target both cognitive variables (e.g., attitudes) and capability (an action-oriented variable) (Malotte et al., 2000). In addition, there must be twice as much increase in the pros than decrease in the cons for behavior change to be supported (Prochaska, Johnson, and Lee, 1998). About 40% of the population with unhealthy behavior is typically at this stage (Fava, Velicer, and Prochaska, 1995).
- *Contemplation* is the stage in which individuals are aware of a problem and are seriously thinking about making a change in the next 6 months, but have not made a commitment to take action. The central element of contemplation is resolving the problem. This entails weighing the pros and cons of the problem and its possible solutions. The cons of changing must also decrease. About 40% of the population with unhealthy behavior is typically at this stage (Fava et al., 1995).
- *Preparation* is a stage that combines intention and behavioral criteria. Individuals in this stage are intending to take action in the next month or have unsuccessfully taken action in the past year. The hallmark of preparation is decision-making. About 20% of the population with unhealthy behavior is typically at this stage (Fava et al., 1995).
- *Action* is the stage in which individuals have modified their behavior, experiences, or environment within the past 6 months in order to overcome their problems.

Modification of the target behavior to an acceptable level and significant overt efforts to change are the hallmarks of action.

- *Maintenance* is the stage when individuals work to prevent relapse and consolidate the gains achieved through action. Stabilizing behavior change and avoiding relapse are the hallmarks of maintenance. Maintenance lasts from 6 months to about 5 years.
- *Termination* is the stage in which individuals have zero temptation to stop the new behavior and 100% capability to continue its use.

Instead of an orderly progression through the stages, relapse and recycling through the stages occur quite frequently. During relapse, individuals regress to an earlier stage.

Steps in the Change Process

Steps in the change process have been adapted from the Transtheoretical model by Bracken, Timmreck, and Church (2001, p. 357). Their streamlined steps are:

1. *Becoming aware*—developing an awareness of the need for change
2. *Preparing for change and development planning*—making the commitment to change, setting goals, and developing a plan of action
3. *Taking action*—doing what it takes to develop new behaviors and discard old ones
4. *Maintaining the gain*—developing processes to maintain the gain

Stages of change have been studied in smoking cessation, stopping cocaine use, weight control, high-fat diets, adolescent delinquent behaviors, safe sex, condom use, sunscreen use, radon gas exposure, exercise acquisition, mammography screening, and physician's preventive practices with smokers (Prochaska, Velicer et al., 1994). One recent longitudinal study of stage transition for exercise found the strongest support in retention of the action/maintenance stage, with limited implications for progression from the precontemplation and preparation stages (Plotnikoff, Hotz, Birkett, and Courneya, 2001). However, using three outcomes in a study of smokers (habit strength, positive evaluation strength, and negative evaluation strength), movement from the stages of precontemplation, contemplation, or preparation was accurately predicted 1 year later, with 36 of the 40 predictions confirmed (Velicer, Norman, Fava, and Prochaska, 1999). Rodgers and colleagues found that the behavioral processes were more sensitive than the cognitive processes for distinguishing between stages of exercise behavior (Rodgers et al., 2001). The most significant implication of stage change research is for the nurse to evaluate each client's readiness for change before attempting any interventions. After an assessment, specific interventions can be tailored to the client's stage of readiness.

Laitakari (1998) suggests that the stage model is realistic and has many positive aspects. This model makes it clear that one learning experience or environmental modification is usually not sufficient for the adoption of a new behavior. A planned series of learning experiences or environmental changes, implemented in an atmosphere of mutual trust, is needed to support the change or adoption process. The nurse must not try to manipulate a client's behavior in a predetermined direction.

Another benefit is a client-centered approach where each individual is assessed and given feedback about their apparent readiness for change, within the context of supportive environmental and social factors. In addition, the stage model provides order and direction to health education and health promotion efforts. Instead of taking the longitudinal process of behavior change for granted, stage-specific experiences can be planned, while respecting the individual's responsibility for independent decision-making. And, finally, the concept of a stage is easy to understand and is seen as meaningful by both clients and professionals.

Behavioral Initiation/Maintenance Stage Theory

Rothman and colleagues (2004) have proposed a stage theory that differentiates behavioral initiation decisions from those made during behavioral maintenance. They suggest that decisions regarding starting a behavior change (behavioral initiation) are based on expected outcomes. Decisions regarding the maintenance of behavior change "involve a consideration of the experiences people have had engaging in the new pattern of behavior and a determination of whether those experiences are sufficiently desirable to warrant continued action" (Rothman, Baldwin, and Hertel, 2004, p. 133). Individuals may choose to continue an initial behavior change plan, modify the plan, suspend the plan briefly or intermittently, and/or discontinue trying to implement the new behavior. In this model, maintenance is viewed as a process rather than as the last step in the behavior change process (Wing, 2000).

The first stage in this theory is the *initial response,* which starts as soon as the behavior change process begins, and lasts until the first significant change is implemented. Self-efficacy and health beliefs are important factors at this stage, which roughly corresponds to the Transtheoretical Model's stages of precontemplation, contemplation, preparation, and action. The second stage is *continued response,* in which the ability and motivation to engage consistently in the new pattern of behavior is challenged by unpleasant experiences that lead to a vulnerability for lapses and relapses. This stage is comparable to the Transtheoretical Model's stage of maintenance. The third stage in this model is *maintenance,* in which there is a desire to sustain the new, successful pattern of behavior. Maintenance may be related to the perceived value of the behavior rather than ability to perform the behavior. The fourth stage is labeled *habit,* where the behavior is self-sustained, comparable to the Transtheoretical Model's stage of termination. This model provides an alternative perspective on processes of change.

Processes of Change

Ten different processes that explain how change occurs have received empirical and theoretical support across various theories (Prochaska, DiClemente, and Norcross, 1992). These processes of change are matched with representative interventions in Table 13-2.

The nurse can match interventions to a client's key characteristics by applying or avoiding particular processes at each stage of change listed below (Jordan & Nigg, 2002; Prochaska, DiClemente, and Norcross, 1992, p. 1109).

- *Precontemplation stage*—clients at this stage use significantly fewer change processes than individuals at the other stages. Precontemplators process less information about problems, devote less time and energy to reevaluation, experience

Table 13-2. Titles, Definitions, and Representative Interventions of the Processes of Change

PROCESS	DEFINITIONS AND INTERVENTIONS
Consciousness raising	Increasing information about self and problem: observations, confrontations, interpretations, bibliotherapy
Self-reevaluation	Assessing how one feels and thinks about oneself with respect to a problem: value clarification, imagery, corrective emotional experience
Self-liberation	Choosing and commitment to act or belief in ability to change: decision-making therapy, New Year's resolutions, logotherapy techniques, commitment-enhancing techniques
Counter-conditioning	Substituting alternatives for problem behaviors: relaxation, desensitization, assertion, positive self-statements
Stimulus control	Avoiding or countering stimuli that elicit problem behaviors: restructuring one's environment (e.g., removing alcohol or fattening foods), avoiding high risk cues, fading techniques
Reinforcement management	Rewarding oneself or being rewarded by others for making changes: contingency contracts, over and covert reinforcement, self-reward
Helping relationships	Being open and trusting about problems with someone who cares: therapeutic alliance, social support, self-help groups
Dramatic relief	Experiencing and expressing feelings about one's problems and solutions: psychodrama, grieving losses, role playing
Environmental reevaluation	Assessing how one's problem affects physical environment: empathy training, documentaries
Social liberation	Increasing alternatives for nonproblem behaviors available in society: advocating for rights of repressed; empowering policy interventions

fewer emotional reactions to the negative aspects of problems, are less open with significant others about problems, and do little to shift their attention or environment in the direction to overcoming problems. The goal is to increase the client's awareness of the need for change by becoming more aware of the pros (e.g., listing 10 pros of the desired behavior), consciousness raising, dramatic relief (e.g., feeling the worry about their risk behavior), and environmental reevaluation (e.g., considering how their behavior may affect their social environment).

- *Contemplation stage*—at this stage clients are very open to consciousness-raising techniques, such as observations, confrontations, and interpretations, and dramatic relief experiences that raise emotions and lower negative affect if change occurs. However, individuals at this stage are often described as ambivalent to change or procrastinators. During this stage clients are more likely to reevaluate their values and problems and their effect on significant others. Nursing interventions should focus on decreasing the cons of the desired behavior by encouraging self-reevaluation (e.g., visualization; role-playing), and social liberation (the awareness of opportunities that exist).

- *Preparation stage*—a transitional stage, where there is less reliance on thinking and more focus on behavior. Nursing interventions should emphasize increasing self-efficacy, helping relationships, self-liberation, stimulus control, and counter-conditioning processes.

- *Action stage*—at this stage clients rely increasingly on support and understanding from helping relationships. They believe that they have autonomy and willpower, but need to be reminded about how far they have come. Nurses need to be aware that clients at this stage are at risk for relapse, so reinforcement management and stimulus control are helpful interventions (e.g., self-reevaluation and self-talk strategies).

- *Maintenance stage*—at this stage it is important to do an assessment of the conditions that promote relapse, and develop alternative (and non–self-defeating) responses. It is vital for clients to see maintaining change as very important to them and to at least one significant other. At this stage the nurse can help the client use self-reevaluation, reinforcement management, and counter-conditioning processes to maintain change.

- *Relapse*—it is important for clients to learn from their setbacks in order to continue making progress.

- *Termination*—at this stage individuals report 100% confidence and zero temptation to revert to prior behavior. This stage may be common in addictions because these behaviors require daily motivation to continue their implementation. This stage is less evident in the acquisition of behaviors, because once a bad habit is removed, it no longer requires attention. Lasting behavior change occurs only after multiple trials and through intermediate steps (Goldstein, DePue, Kazura, and Niaura, 1998).

Decisional Balance

Part of the decision to move toward action is believed to be based on the relative weight given to the pros and cons of changing behavior. According to Prochaska, Redding,

Harlow, Rossi, and Velicer (1994), the pros, incentives, or perceived benefits are advantages or positive aspects of changing behavior (i.e., facilitators of change). The cons or perceived barriers to action are the disadvantages or negative aspects of changing behavior (i.e., barriers to change).

Benefits and barriers of behavior change have been incorporated into at least six multidimensional models of health behavior (Leddy, 1997). Perceived barriers were found to be the most powerful dimension of the Health Belief Model (Becker, Haefner, Kasl, Kirscht, Maiman, and Rosenstock, 1977) in explaining various health behaviors (Janz & Becker, 1984). And the advantages of behavior change outweighed the disadvantages as one of eight critical variables in the Theory of Reasoned Action (Fishbein & Ajzen, 1975; Fishbein, Bandura, Triandis, Kanfer, and Becker, 1991). Benefits and barriers are empirically supported as predictors of health behaviors in the majority of studies using the Health Promotion Model (Pender, 1996), with barriers receiving the strongest support and benefits receiving moderate support. Pros and cons are variables in the Health Behavior Change model (Leddy, 2004. In the Transtheoretical model (Prochaska & DiClemente, 1984), incentives (i.e., pros) accounted for more of the variance in the movement through behavior change stages, whereas barriers (i.e., cons) remained relatively stable across the stages of change (Prochaska, Redding et al., 1994). Consequently, there may be more openness for nursing interventions to increase incentives rather than to decrease barriers to behavior change. Measures of decisional balance also have demonstrated predictive utility for smoking cessation (Prochaska, DiClemente, Velicer, Ginpil, and Norcross, 1985) and exercise readiness (Marcus & Owen, 1992) in studies based on the Multiattribute Utility Theory (Carter, 1990).

A meta-analysis of 24 retrospective studies demonstrated a significantly large effect for both benefits and barriers for health-related behaviors (Harrison, Mullen, and Green, 1992). As most behavior change will relapse (Prochaska, Redding et al., 1994), it is desirable for nursing interventions to focus on increasing the incentives as well as trying to decrease the barriers for health behavior change.

Self-Efficacy

Bandura (1977) developed the concept of self-efficacy to describe how capable an individual feels about performing specific tasks in specific behavioral situations. Self-efficacy theory proposes that confidence in the ability to perform a given behavior is strongly related to the actual ability to perform the behavior. Outcome expectancies are related to judgments individuals make regarding their ability to use skills necessary to carry out the behavior. In contrast, self-efficacy affects judgments of the probable consequences of a certain behavior (Holloway & Watson, 2002). Although the individual's efficacy expectations will vary greatly depending on the particular task and context, perceived self-efficacy is believed to influence all aspects of behavior (Strecher, DeVellis, Becker, and Rosenstock, 1986) including:

- *Acquisition of new behaviors* (e.g., a sexually-active young adult learning how to use a particular contraceptive device)
- *Inhibition of existing behaviors* (e.g., decreasing or stopping cigarette smoking)
- *Disinhibition of behaviors* (e.g., resuming sexual activity after a heart attack)

- *Choices of behavioral settings*
- *Amount of effort expended on a task*
- *Length of time spent persisting in the face of obstacles*
- *Emotional reactions* (e.g., anxiety and distress)
- *Thought patterns* (e.g., ruminating about personal deficiencies rather than thinking about accomplishing a task)

According to Bandura (1977), efficacy expectations vary in magnitude (ordering of tasks by difficulty), strength (certainty of ability to perform a task), and generality (degree to which expectations about one task apply to other tasks). In addition, Bandura, O'Leary, Taylor, Gauthier, and Gossard (1987) have linked the judgment of capability to perform with the perceived ability to exercise control over events. In a modification of Bandura's concept, the Transtheoretical model views self-efficacy as both confidence in changing a problem behavior, and resistance to situational temptation to engage in the problem behavior (Prochaska, Redding et al., 1994).

"Manipulations of self-efficacy have proved influential in attempts to initiate and modify health behaviors" (Holloway & Watson, 2002, p. 112). Marcus, Selby, Niaura, and Rossi (1992) found that exercise self-efficacy was significantly related to stage in the change process. Individuals at the precontemplation stage scored the lowest in self-efficacy and those at the maintenance stage scored the highest. Plotnikoff and colleagues (2001), in a longitudinal study, also found moderate to strong support of exercise self-efficacy as a predictor of moving ahead to the next stage. In smoking cessation studies, confidence is an important predictor of stage movement to action and maintenance, while temptation is an important predictor of relapse (Prochaska, Redding et al., 1994). Self-efficacy has been shown to be related to many other health behaviors, including contraceptive behavior, cardiac rehabilitation, weight loss, and nutrition (AbuSabha & Achterberg, 1997). Increased self-efficacy in clients with cancer has also been associated with increased adherence to treatment, increased self-care behaviors, and decreased symptoms (Lev, 1997).

Locus of Control

Locus of control is often confused with self-efficacy. Locus of control is based on an individual's view of their ability to achieve a particular outcome. They either see control as internal, where their actions determine the outcome, or they see control as outside of themselves where reward is controlled by external forces (Rotter, 1954). Levenson (1974) extended external beliefs into two beliefs that include chance expectations (fate or luck) and control by powerful others (family members or physicians). Whereas self-efficacy is task specific, locus of control is more general and is believed to be domain specific (e.g., health domain, social domain). However, locus of control has limited stability across time or different domains.

Studies have shown that individuals with an "internal" locus of control take responsibility for their actions and engage more readily in health-promoting behaviors (AbuSabha & Achterberg, 1997). However, when used alone, the effect of locus of control on behavior is small. Wallston (1992, p. 194) suggests "a rapprochement" (reconciliation) of Rotter's and Bandura's social learning theories, substituting a generalized expectancy of control for locus of control, and incorporating perceived competence. The revised view states that "people must value health as an outcome, believe that their health actions influence their health status, and concurrently believe that they are capable of carrying out the necessary behaviors in order to have a high likelihood of engaging in a health-directed action" (Wallston, 1992, p. 195). A study of ten health behaviors in 4358 female and 2757 male university students from 18 European countries showed that high chance locus scores were associated with 20% to 35% reductions in the likelihood of healthy options for six of the behaviors. This seems to indicate when chance or fate are seen as controlling factors there is a reduction in the possibility of the healthy behavior actually occurring. For several of the behaviors associated with internal locus of control, the odds of carrying out healthy activities were 40% to 70% greater for those in the highest quartile for internal locus of control, compared with the lowest quartile (Steptoe & Wardle, 2001). The perceived health competence concept appears to hold promise as a predictor of adherence behavior (Christensen, Wiebe, Benotsch, and Lawton, 1996).

Health Beliefs

A belief is the conviction of truth (or falsehood) of an association between two concepts. A belief may be based on observation. For example, feeling energized after exercise would support the belief that exercise increases vitality. Scientific evidence may also support a belief, such as research supporting a link between exercise and reduction of myocardial disease. Some of the specific health beliefs that have been found to influence behavior include:

- *Perceived susceptibility*—the belief of being vulnerable to a particular health problem
- *Perceived severity*—the belief that a health problem has potential serious consequences
- *Perceived consequences* (also called outcome expectations)—beliefs regarding the consequences (positive or negative) of performing a specific health behavior
- *Perceived benefits*—the belief that taking action toward improving health will prevent illness or improve health
- *Value of health*—a measurement of the importance placed on outcome expectations
- *Perceived barriers*—the belief that certain personal or environmental factors make it difficult/impossible to take action toward improving health behavior
- *Perceived threat*—a combination of personal susceptibility and seriousness of a particular health problem
- *Perceived self-efficacy*—how capable the individual feels about performing a specific task in a specific behavioral situation

Health beliefs are incorporated into a number of health behavior models. Beliefs are the fundamental building blocks in the Theory of Reasoned Action, as "the totality of a person's beliefs serves as the informational base that ultimately determines his attitudes, intentions, and behaviors" (Fishbein & Ajzen, 1975, p. 14). However, in a review of 10 years of studies related to the Health Belief Model (Rosenstock, 1966), Janz and Becker

(1984) concluded that only two of the belief components, perceived barriers and perceived susceptibility, explained or predicted preventive behaviors.

The revised Health Promotion Model (Pender, Murdaugh, and Parsons, 2002) has been proposed as a "third generation model" that focuses specifically on health decisions and the resulting behavior. This model attempts to combine decision analysis, behavioral decision theory, and health beliefs. Other variables that are incorporated are efficacy, assessment of the importance of good health, and 'cues to action' that apply specifically to the client-caregiver interaction (Clark & Becker, 1998). Studies of the earlier Health Promotion Model (Pender, 1996) support the impact of perceived benefits and perceived self-efficacy in addition to perceived barriers on behavior.

Other Influences on Health Behavior

Pender, Murdaugh, and Parsons (2002), in the revised Health Promotion Model (HPM), have proposed a complex combination of individual characteristics and experiences, behavior-specific thinking, and behavioral outcomes. Other influences affecting health behavior include:

- *Prior related behavior*—having performed the same or a similar behavior in the past
- *Personal factors*—prediction of behavior is shaped by the nature of the target behavior
- *Activity-related affect*—subjective feelings before, during, and after a behavior
- *Interpersonal influences*—thoughts concerning behaviors, beliefs, or attitudes of others
- *Situational influences*—perceptions and thoughts about the context for behavior
- *Commitment to a plan of action*—intent to carry out a specific action including planned strategies
- *Competing demands and preferences*—alternative behaviors that become competing courses of action to an intended health-promoting behavior

Support has previously been found for many of the behavior-specific cognitions, including perceived benefits, perceived self-efficacy, and perceived barriers (Pender, 1996). The variables of activity-related affect, commitment to a plan of action, and immediate competing demands and preferences are new variables. The entire revised model is undergoing testing.

The Health Behavior Goal Model

The behavior goal model integrates aspects of expectancy, value, stage, and goal theories. "The model's features are that it (1) incorporates the personal goal structure of the individual, (2) encompasses phases of change, (3) focuses on individual emotional and health costs as well as benefits of changing the behavior, (4) takes into account an individual's perception of his or her own capacities, as well as the perceived influence of the direct environment, and (5) recognizes personal as well as environmental sources of change" (Moes & Gebhardt, 2000, p. 365).

The probability of adoption of a target health behavior is higher when it is specific (the nature of the behavior is important), seen as important, and relatively easy to attain within a reasonable period of time. The expected consequences of the target health behavior are divided into (1) perceived health costs and benefits, (2) perceived emotional costs and benefits, (3) social influence (the individual's appraisal of how the social environment would react to adoption of the target health behavior), and (4) perceived competence (the assessment of an individual's capacity to execute the behavior). The process of change is assumed to occur through certain distinct, sequential stages. During each of these stages, relapse is possible.

This chapter continues in Chapter 14, in which multicultural competency and behavior change interventions are discussed.

References

AbuSabha, R., & Achterberg, C. (1997). Review of self-efficacy and locus of control for nutrition- and health-related behavior. *Journal of the American Dietetic Association, 97,* 1122–1132.

Ajzen, I. (1985). From intentions to actions: A theory of planned behavior. In J. Kuhl & J. Beckmann (Eds.), *Action-control: From cognition to behavior* (pp. 11–39). Hidelberg: Springer.

Bandura, A. (1977). Self-efficacy: Toward a unifying theory of behavioral change. *Psychological Review, 84,* 191–215.

Bandura, A. (1986). *Social foundations of thought and action: A social cognitive theory.* Englewood Cliffs, NJ: Prentice-Hall.

Bandura, A., O'Leary, A., Taylor, C. B., Gauthier, J., & Gossard, D. (1987). Perceived self-efficacy and pain control: Opioid and non-opioid mechanisms. *Journal of Personality and Social Psychology, 53,* 563–571.

Becker, M. H., Haefner, D. P., Kasl, S. V., Kirscht, J. P., Maiman, L. A., & Rosenstock, I. M. (1977). Selected psychosocial models and correlates of individual health-related behaviors. *Medical Care, 15*(Suppl.), 27–46.

Boekaerts, M., Pintrich, P. R., & Zeidner, M. (2000). *Handbook of self-regulation.* San Diego, CA: Academic Press.

Bracken, D. W., Timmreck, C. W., & Church, A. H. (2001). *The handbook of multisource feedback: The comprehensive resource for designing and implementing MSF processes.* San Francisco: Jossey-Bass.

Cameron, L. D., & Leventhal, H. (2002). Self-regulation, health and illness. In L. D. Cameron & H. Leventhal (Eds.), *The self-regulation of health and illness behavior* (pp. 1–13). London: Routledge.

Carter, W. B. (1990). Health behavior as a rational process: Theory of reasoned action and multiattribute utility theory. In K. Glanz, F. M. Lewis, & B. K. Rimer (Eds.), *Health behavior and health education* (pp. 63–91). San Francisco: Jossey-Bass.

Christensen, A. J., Wiebe, J. S., Benotsch, E. G., & Lawton, W. J. (1996). Perceived health competence, health locus of control, and patient adherence in renal dialysis. *Cognitive Therapy and Research, 20,* 411–421.

Clark, N. M., & Becker, M. H. (1998). Theoretical models and strategies for improving adherence and disease management. In S. A. Schumaker, E. B. Schron, J. K. Oksene, & W. L. McBee (Eds.), *The handbook of human behavior change* (2nd ed., pp. 5–32). New York: Springer.

Fava, J. L., Velicer, W. F., & Prochaska, J. O. (1995). Applying the transtheoretical model to a representative sample of smokers. *Addictive Behaviors, 20,* 189–203.

Fishbein, M., & Ajzen, I. (1975). *Belief, attitude, intention and behavior: An introduction to theory and research.* Reading, MA: Addison-Wesley.

Fishbein, M., Bandura, A., Triandis, H. C., Kanfer, F., & Becker, M. (1991). Factors influencing behavior and behavior change: Final report of theorist's workshop on AIDS-related behaviors. Washington DC: National Institute of Mental Health, National Institutes of Health.

Goldstein, M. G., DePue, J., Kazura, A., & Niaura, R. (1998). Models for provider-patient interaction: Applications to health behavior change. In S. A. Schumaker, E. B. Schron, J. K. Ockene, & W. L. McBee (Eds.), *The handbook of health behavior change* (2nd ed.). New York: Springer.

Harrison, J. A., Mullen, P. D., & Green, L. W. (1992). A meta-analysis of studies of the health belief model with adults. *Health Education Research, 7,* 107–116.

Holloway, A., & Watson, H. E. (2002). Role of self-efficacy and behavior change. *International Journal of Nursing Practice, 8,* 106–115.

Janz, N. K., & Becker, M. H. (1984). The health belief model: A decade later. *Health Education Quarterly, 11(1),* 1–47.

Jeffery, R. W., Drewnowski, A., Epstein, L. H., Stunkard, A. J., Wilson, G. T., Wing, R. R., & Hill, R. (2000). Long-term maintenance of weight loss: Current status. *Health Psychology, 19*(Suppl.), 5–16.

Jordan, P. J., & Nigg, C. R. (2002). Applying the transtheoretical model: Tailoring interventions to stages of change. In P. M. Burbank & D. Reibe. *Promoting exercise and behavior change in older adults: Interventions with the transtheoretical model.* New York: Springer.

Kumanyika, S. K., Van Horn, L., Bowen, D., Perri, M. G., Rolls, B. J., Czajkowski, S. M., & Schron, I. (2000). Maintenance on dietary behavior change. *Health Psychology, 19*(Suppl.), 42–56.

Laitakari, J. (1998). On the practical applicability of stage models to health promotion and health education. *American Journal of Health Behavior, 22,* 28–38.

Leddy, S. K. (1996). Development and psychometric testing of the Leddy Healthiness Scale. *Research in Nursing and Health, 19,* 431–440.

Leddy, S. K. (1997). Incentives and barriers to exercise in women with a history of breast cancer. *Oncology Nursing Forum, 24,* 885–890.

Leddy, S. K. (2004). The health behavior change model. Unpublished manuscript.

Lev, E. L. (1997). Bandura's theory of self-efficacy: Applications to oncology. *Scholarly Inquiry for Nursing Practice, 11(1),* 21–37.

Levenson, H. (1974). Activism and powerful others: Distinctions within the concept of internal-external control. *Journal of Personality Assessment, 38,* 377–383.

Leventhal, H., Meyer, D., & Nerenz, D. (1980). The common sense representation of illness danger. In S. Rachman (Ed.), *Contributions to medical psychology* (pp. 7–30). New York: Pergamon Press.

Malotte, C. K., Jarvis, B., Fishbein, M., Kamb, M., Iatesta, M., Hoxworth, T., Zenilman, J., Bolan, G., & the Project RESPECT Study Group (2000). State of change versus an integrated psychosocial theory as a basis for developing effective behavior change interventions. *AIDS Care, 12,* 357–364.

Marcus, B. H., & Owen, N. (1992). Motivational readiness, self-efficacy and decision-making for exercise. *Journal of Applied Social Psychology, 22(1),* 3–16.

Marcus, B. H., Selby, V. C., Niaura, R. S., & Rossi, J. S. (1992). Self-efficacy and the stages of exercise behavior change. *Research Quarterly for Exercise and Sport, 63,* 60–66.

Marcus, B. H., Dubbert, P. M., Forsyth, L. H., McKenzie, T. L., Stone, E. J., Dunn, A. L., & Blair, S. N. (2000). Physical activity behavior change: Issues in adoption and maintenance. *Health Psychology, 19*(Suppl.), 32–41.

Moes, S., & Gebhardt, W. (2000). Self-regulation and health behavior: The health behavior goal model. In M. Boekaerts, P. R. Pintrich, & M. Zeidner (Eds.), *Handbook of self-regulation* (pp. 343–363). San Diego, CA: Academic Press.

O'Hea, E. L., Wood, K. B., & Brantley, P. J. (2003). The transtheoretical model: Gender differences across 3 health behaviors. *American Journal of Health Behavior, 27,* 645–656.

Orleans, C. T. (2000). Promoting the maintenance of health behavior change: Recommendations for the next generation of research and practice. *Health Psychology, 19*(Suppl.), 76–83.

Pender, N. J. (1996). *Health promotion in nursing practice* (3rd ed.). Stamford, CT: Appleton & Lange.

Pender, N. J., Murdaugh, C. J., & Parsons, M. A. (2002). *Health promotion in nursing practice* (4th ed.). Upper Saddle River, NJ: Prentice-Hall.

Plotnikoff, R. C., Hotz, S. B., Birkett, N. J., & Courneya, K. S. (2001). Exercise and the transtheoretical model: A longitudinal test of a population sample. *Preventive Medicine, 33,* 441–452.

Prochaska, J. O., & DiClemente, C. C. (1984). *The transtheoretical approach: Crossing traditional boundaries of change.* Homewood, IL: Dow Jones-Irwin.

Prochaska, J. O., DiClemente, C. C., & Norcross, J. C. (1992). In search of how people change. *American Psychologist, 47,* 1102–1114.

Prochaska, J. O., DiClemente, C. C., Velicer, W. F., Ginpil, S., & Norcross, J. C. (1985). Predicting change in smoking status for self-changers. *Addictive Behavior, 10,* 395–406.

Prochaska, J. O., Johnson, S., & Lee, P. (1998). The Transtheoretical model of behavior change. In S. A. Schumaker, E. B. Schron, J. K. Ockene, & W. L. McBee. (Eds.), *The handbook of health behavior change* (2nd ed., pp. 59–84). New York: Springer.

Prochaska, J. O., Redding, C. A., Harlow, L. L., Rossi, J. S., & Velicer, W. F. (1994). The transtheoretical model of change and HIV prevention: A review. *Health Education Quarterly, 21,* 471–486.

Prochaska, J. O., Velicer, W. F., Rossi, J. S., Goldstein, M. G., Marcus, B., Rakowski, et al. (1994). Stages of change and decisional balance for 12 problem behaviors. *Health Psychology, 13,* 39–46.

Quackenbush, R. L. (2001). Comparison and contrast between belief system theory and cognitive theory. *The Journal of Psychology, 123,* 315–328.

Rodgers, W. M., Courneya, K. S., & Bayduza, A. L. (2001). Examination of the transtheoretical model and exercise in 3 populations. *American Journal of Health Behavior, 25,* 33–41.

Rosenstock, I. M. (1966, July). Why people use health services. *Milbank Memorial Fund Quarterly, 44,* 94–127.

Rosenstock, I. M., Strecher, V. J., & Becker, M. H. (1988). Social learning theory and the health belief model. *Health Education Quarterly, 15,* 175–183.

Rothman, A. J., Baldwin, A. S., & Hertel, A. W. (2004). Self-regulation and behavior change: Disentangling behavioral initiation and behavioral maintenance. In R. F. Baumeister & K. D. Vohs (Eds.), *Handbook of self-regulation: Research, theory, and applications* (pp. 130–148). New York: Guilford.

Rotter, J. B. (1954). *Social learning and clinical psychology* (Vol. 80). Englewood Cliffs, NJ: Prentice-Hall.

Steptoe, A., & Wardle, J. (2001). Locus of control and health behaviour revisited: A multivariate analysis of young adults from 18 countries. *British Journal of Psychology, 92,* 659–672.

Strecher, V. J., DeVellis, B. M., Becker, M. H., & Rosenstock, I. M. (1986). The role of self-efficacy in achieving health behavior change. *Health Education Quarterly, 13,* 73–91.

Velicer, W. F., Norman, G. J., Fava, J. L., & Prochaska, J. O. (1999). Testing 40 predictions from the transtheoretical model. *Addictive Behavior, 24,* 455–469.

Wallston, K. A. (1992). Hocus-pocus, the focus isn't strictly on locus: Rotter's social learning theory modified for health. *Cognitive Therapy and Research, 16,* 183–199.

Wallston, K. A., Maides, S. A., & Wallston, B. S. (1976). Health related information seeking as a function of health related locus of control and health value. *Journal of Research in Personality, 10,* 215–222.

Wing, R. R. (2000). Cross-cutting themes in maintenance of behavior change. *Health Psychology, 19,* 84–88.

CHAPTER 14

Health Behavior Change Interventions

Concepts
Ethnocentric Monoculturalism

Figures & Tables
Table 14-1 Nursing Interventions by Stages of Change

Models and Theories
Systems Model of Clinical Preventive Care
Transtheoretical Model Processes of Change
Motivational Interviewing
Brief Negotiation Model
Patient-Centered Counseling Model
Relapse Prevention

Helpful Lists
Implications of Cultural Competency, pgs. 174–175
Barriers Affecting Education and Counseling, pgs. 177–178
Caregiver False Assumptions, pg. 178
Resistance to Changing Behavior, pg. 179
Motivational Interviewing Behaviors, pg. 183
Principles of Motivational Interviewing, pg. 183
Strategies for Behavior Change, pgs. 183–184
Principles for the Brief Negotiation Model, pg. 184
Suggestions for Behavior Change Interventions, pg. 187

Thought Questions
1. What are the elements to consider for church-based health promotion? How can the nurse intervene effectively in these areas?
2. Can you identify five ways in which the nurse can promote client health behavior change?
3. Think about the list of false assumptions you may hold. How can you change your incorrect beliefs?
4. How can organizational barriers to implementing individual behavior change in an institutional setting (e.g., hospitals) be overcome?
5. How can the nurse address client resistance to changing health behavior? Can you explain the rationale for your choices?
6. Do you think that social and environmental policy levels are appropriate for nursing interventions? Why or why not? Can you see yourself implementing "upstream" strategies?

Chapter Synopsis

This chapter provides an in-depth discussion of intervention strategies to promote individual behavior change. Many of the strategies involve feedback, behavior modification, providing information, reinforcement, and ways to enhance the nurse-client relationship. A number of models for intervention are reviewed, including the systems model of clinical preventive care, the Transtheoretical Model processes of change, motivational interviewing, the brief negotiation model, and the patient-centered counseling model. Relapse prevention is discussed in depth. Finally, it is becoming increasingly clear that maintenance of long-term behavior change requires multiple level, linked, interpersonal, community, environmental, and health-care system approaches as well as individual interventions.

MULTICULTURAL COMPETENCY

Racism continues to be a source of stress in the lives of individuals of color. They are subjected to prejudice, bias, and discrimination in education, housing, and employment and are more likely to live in poverty (Sue, 2002). High proportions of minorities are medically uninsured, but are less likely to be insured by Medicaid, and/or live in medically underserved areas. Unfortunately, public health practices are often culturally inappropriate and antagonistic to the lifestyles and values of minority groups.

Ethnocentric Monoculturalism

Often members of different groups believe their cultural heritage is superior to that of other cultures. This belief may be evident in the group's collective history, values, language, traditions, or arts and crafts. Sometimes, members of health-care professions may feel that their way of doing things is the "best way," revealing conscious or unconscious feelings of superiority. Because western science guides health-care practice it is often considered a "superior" form of treatment, resulting in indigenous forms of treatment being consigned to an "inferior and unscientific" status (Sue, 2002). When the health-care treatment of another culture is seen as inferior there is a tendency to view the entire culture, including its customs, values, traditions, and language this way. This belief can result in the dominant group imposing their standards and beliefs on a less powerful group or culture.

Cultural Competency

Cultural competency has implications for all health-care providers. When learning to become more culturally competent, it is important for the nurse to:

1. Become culturally aware of personal values, biases, and assumptions about human behavior.
2. Acquire knowledge and understanding of the worldview of clients, especially those from minority or culturally different groups.
3. Begin the process of developing culturally appropriate and effective health-care interventions by working with culturally different clients and communities.

4. Begin to understand how organizational and institutional forces can enhance or negate the development of multicultural competency. It is possible for hospitals, insurance carriers, and both public and private agencies to actively discourage, negate, or punish multicultural expressions.

"Among Asian and many Asian American groups, for example, a helping relationship is characterized by the following attributes: (1) subtlety and indirectness in communications, (2) vertical or hierarchical communication patterns, (3) respect for authority figures, and (4) the giving of advice and directions by a perceived expert" (Sue, 2002, p. 45). Many Asian American clients expect the nurse to give advice and suggestions, avoid direct interpretation of motives and actions, circumvent confrontation, indirectly discuss personal issues, do more initial talking than the client, and use a formal interaction approach (Sue, 2002). In a study of indigenous healing in 16 nonwestern countries, it was found there is heavy reliance on the use of communal, group, and family networks to shelter the disturbed individual (Saudi Arabia), to problem-solve in a group context (Nigeria), and to reconnect the individual with family or significant others (Korea). In these cultures, spiritual and religious beliefs and traditions of the community are often used in the healing process, and shamans (piris in Pakistan and fakirs in Sudan), are considered the keepers of timeless wisdom.

Church-Based Health Promotion

Church-based health promotion (CBHP) "is a large-scale effort by the church community to improve the health of its members through any combination of education, screening, referral, treatment, and group support" (Peterson, Atwood, and Yates, 2002, p. 402). A literature review identified seven elements that are important for CBHP to address: partnerships, positive health values, availability of services, access to church facilities, community-focused interventions, health behavior change, and supportive social relationships and networks (Peterson et al., 2002). The church has historically served as an advocate, encourager, and supporter of actions on behalf of the underserved, oppressed, and marginalized members of society. The African American church has been especially noteworthy in these respects. Frequently, churches are the center of social, political, and educational functions and are available in almost every community. The structural facilities of churches make them ideal for holding meetings, educational programs, exercise sessions, serving meals, day care, and other activities designed to reach out and serve the community.

ASSESSMENT

An assessment in health behavior change evaluates the importance (based on values) of the behavior change to the client; the client's confidence and feelings of self-efficacy to change behavior; and the client's readiness to make a specific behavior change. There are a number of available instruments to measure confidence, self-efficacy, and readiness for change. If any of these elements is lacking, a number of intervention strategies are available to bolster the client's readiness for sustainable behavior change.

INTERVENTIONS FOR BEHAVIOR CHANGE

Health-related behaviors are either protective in nature (e.g., exercise, good nutrition, and stress management), or negatively impact health (e.g., smoking, drinking, and sedentary lifestyle). It is a challenge for nurses to learn how to help clients adopt and sustain healthy attitudes and habits. "There are no miracle drugs available for helping people change long-standing patterns of living. Simply telling people to stop smoking, eat less fat, have safe sex, exercise more, discontinue their abusive practices, or reduce their life stresses seldom works" (Westberg & Jason, 1996, p. 146). Clients often do not follow the advice of nurses or physicians, particularly when authoritarian "orders" are given. Clients must be actively involved as collaborative partners in assessing their health and developing and monitoring their own long-term health plans. The health professional can best promote and sustain change by educating, supporting, and advising clients.

Interventions for behavior change utilize a number of strategies, including feedback, behavior modification, information, reinforcement, and enhancing the nurse-client relationship. These strategies are discussed in the next section.

Feedback

There are five types of feedback that can be understood along a continuum, with generic feedback at one end, and targeted feedback at the other. *Generic feedback* simply offers the client relevant information that is true for the population the individual belongs to (e.g., the health benefits of exercise). *Personalized feedback* is based on personal information provided by the client. *Targeted feedback* tailors information to some important but still rather general characteristics of the client (e.g., providing information to women over 50 about the importance of mammograms). *Tailored feedback* and *interpersonal feedback* are in ascending order of individualization and assessment, becoming increasingly tailored to the individual and more detailed in providing information specific to the individual. "Most feedback is directed to providing information, critical aspects of attitudes and beliefs about susceptibility, severity, norms, and efficacy, benefits, or barriers that can facilitate changing risk or adopting protective health behaviors" (DiClemente, Marinilli, Singh, and Bellino, 2001, pp. 219–221). At a minimum, feedback heightens the relevance of the message for the client drawing them into interaction with the information.

Behavior Modification

Behavior modification "emphasizes the roles played by habit and skill in attempts to modify undesirable personal (or 'lifestyle') behaviors" (Clark & Becker, 1998, p. 21). This approach frequently follows these steps: (1) identify the problem and describe it in behavioral terms; (2) select a target behavior that is measurable; (3) identify the antecedents and consequences of the behavior; (4) set behavioral objectives; (5) devise and implement a behavior-change program; and (6) evaluate the program.

Providing Information

A number of studies have identified factors associated with the failure to follow therapeutic recommendations. These factors include *poor recall* (after 5 minutes clients forget one-half of the clinician's instructions), recall according to the timing of messages (material presented in the first third of the discussion is best remembered), *selective recall* (clients recall a diagnosis better than therapy recommendations). Recall can be enhanced through labeling and categorizing messages (simple reorganization of a list of 15 medical statements into labeled categories enhanced recall by 50%), and through recognition (well-organized messages repeated several times in a simple leaflet significantly improved adherence to a weight-loss plan) (Clark & Becker, 1998).

Modifying and Reinforcing Elements of the Treatment Experience

Rates of adhering to treatment tend to be lower when the therapeutic regimen is complex, of long duration, dependent on alteration of the client's lifestyle, inconvenient, or expensive. Therapeutic complexity can be simplified by stressing the importance of following through with the critical aspects of the treatment ("prioritizing the regimen"); by breaking the treatment plan into less complex sequential stages; and by minimizing both inconvenience and forgetfulness by matching the regimen schedule to the client's regular activities ("tailoring the regimen"). Client behavior change skills (like all skills) deteriorate over time if not reinforced by use. Clients must know how to determine if the medical regimen is working and be able to identify signs of an emergency situation, should it occur (Clark & Becker, 1998).

In a contingency contract, both parties create a treatment goal, detail the specific obligations of the client and the nurse in reaching the goal, and set a time limit for its achievement. Contracts have a number of benefits including providing a written outline of expected behavior, involving the client in the decision-making process about the regimen and providing an opportunity to discuss potential problems and solutions. Contracts help clients make a formal commitment to the program by providing rewards and incentives, (e.g., additional time spent with the nurse or lottery tickets), which can increase motivation to achieve goals (Clark & Becker, 1998). The family can enhance supervision of the client, as well as provide assistance and encouragement.

Enhancing the Nurse-Client Relationship

Many health-care providers rely on simply providing advice because of inadequate knowledge of effective client education and counseling techniques, such as checking for understanding, addressing feelings about change, enhancing motivation, and negotiating a plan (Goldstein, DePue, Kazura, and Niaura, 1998). Barriers that can affect nursing involvement in client education and counseling are described

1. Deficits in knowledge
2. Deficits in interviewing and assessment skills needed to make an adequate diagnosis of the client's health education needs

3. Deficits in the skills necessary to motivate and assist the clients with behavior change
4. Deficits in the skills necessary to help the client maintain the new behaviors and adhere to the treatment plan
5. Attitudinal barriers
6. Organizational barriers, such as limited reimbursement for counseling and preventive-care services, lack of self-help or other client education resources, poor coordination with behavioral treatment programs or other referral resources, and limited involvement of staff in client education and health-promotion activities
7. Clients feel they are wasting the nurse's valuable time
8. Clients omit details they consider unimportant
9. Clients are embarrassed to mention things they think will place them in an unfavorable light
10. Clients do not understand medical terms
11. Clients may not believe they have really been listened to and therefore assume the nurse does not have the necessary information to make a good treatment decision

The following are false assumptions that may be held by the nurse: (Rollnick, Mason, and Butler, 1999, pp. 34–35)

1. This client OUGHT to change. Fact: Change depends on the client and their perceived need for change, not whether the nurse thinks it is important.
2. This client WANTS to change. Fact: Clients often have conflicting motives and feelings about making a change.
3. The client's health is the prime motivating factor. Fact: There may be other factors that provide greater motivation for change. The nurse can help clients discern their motives and act on them effectively. Health doesn't have to be the prime motivator for a client to make a healthy change.
4. If the client does not decide to change, the consultation has failed. Fact: Deciding to change is a process, not an event, and it takes time.
5. Clients are either motivated to change, or not. Fact: The motivation to do something is not an all-or-nothing phenomenon; it is a matter of degree.
6. Now is the right time to consider change. Fact: But it might not be the best time for the client.
7. A tough approach is always best. Fact: Most clients do not respond well to authoritative communication, which can result in the client resisting change.
8. The nurse is the expert and the client must follow the advice given. Fact: Telling the client what to do does not encourage behavior change. When clients are equal partners in their care they are more willing to take responsibility for change.

Communication is improved when the health-care provider focuses on the treatment plan, has a congenial demeanor, and uses reassuring communication (Clark & Becker, 1998). Other strategies include being attentive to the client; eliciting the client's underlying concerns about the condition; addressing immediate concerns expressed by the client by engaging in interactive conversation via open-ended questions, using simple language and analogies to teach important concepts; tailoring the regimen by eliciting and addressing potential problems in the timing, dosage, or side effects of medications; using appropriate nonverbal encouragement and verbal praise when the client reports using correct disease-management strategies; constructing reassuring messages that alleviate fears; eliciting the client's immediate objective and reaching an agreement with the patient and the family on short-term goals; reviewing the long-term plan for treatment so the client knows what to expect over time and understands the situations under which the physician will modify treatment, and knows the criteria for judging the success of the treatment plan; and helping the client plan in advance for making decisions about their condition.

INTERVENTION MODELS

A Systems Model of Clinical Preventive Care

According to Walsh and McPhee's (1992) model, both the client and health provider have *predisposing* factors (cognitive, attitudinal, and perceptual), *enabling* factors (skills and resources necessary to perform the behavior), and *reinforcing* factors (skills and resources that support or reward the preventive activity) that influence their willingness to engage in health behavior change. The model recognizes other factors that independently influence both the physician (or nurse) and the client, including health-care delivery/organizational factors, preventive activity factors, and situational factors/cues to action. If these client or provider factors are considered independently, the content of the interaction is not emphasized, and the process of the interaction is not considered (Goldstein et al., 1998). Therefore, the model emphasizes the *mutual* nurse-client interaction.

The idea of changing health behavior is often uncomfortable. Deeply ingrained habits, even harmful ones are often difficult to change and most clients find it hard to make even minor changes. According to Westberg and Jason (1996), individuals tend to resist change because of beliefs that changing their behavior may:

- Require giving up pleasure (e.g., eating high-fat ice cream)
- Be unpleasant (e.g., doing certain exercises)
- Be overtly painful (e.g., discontinuing addictive substances)
- Be stressful (e.g., facing social situations without alcohol)
- Jeopardize social relationships (e.g., engaging in unprotected adolescent sex)
- Not seem important anymore (e.g., in the case of older individuals)
- Require alteration in self-image (e.g., in the case of a hard-working executive learning how to play)

These beliefs and fears can make it difficult to change long-standing habits and attitudes.

Transtheoretical Model Processes of Change

According to Prochaska, Velicer, Rossi, Goldstein, Marcus, Rakowski et al. (1994), some of the most frequently used strategies to help clients modify their behavior include consciousness raising, self-reevaluation, environmental reevaluation, self-liberation, social liberation, helping relationships, stimulus control, counterconditioning, and reinforcement management. These strategies and techniques have been linked with movement along the stages of change in the Transtheoretical Model. Other intervention strategies organized by the stages of the Transtheoretical Model are indicated in Table 14-1, which is adapted from Miller and Rollnick (1991).

Table 14-1. **Stages of Change**

STAGE	NURSING INTERVENTIONS
Precontemplation Stage Goal—Client begins to think about making a change.	· Provide information over time in small amounts. · Use teachable moments, for example, using the symptoms as a message. · Ask questions. For example, "If you decided to make a change what might be some of the advantages?"
Contemplation Stage Goal—Client examines advantages of and barriers to change.	· Find out what the client thinks are reasons to change, and barriers to change. · Restate both sides of any ambivalence. · Brainstorm on solutions for one barrier at a time.
Preparation Stage Goal—Client considers actions necessary to begin to make a change.	· Ask the client for a goal date to begin making a change. · Continue to support and encourage the client's efforts to change.
Action Stage Goal—Client takes decisive actions.	· Reinforce the client's decisions. · Express appreciation for even small successes. · Ask what else can be done to ensure success.
Maintenance Stage Goal—Change is added to the client's daily life.	· Continue to encourage and positively reinforce client's change. · Ask what strategies have been helpful and what situations continue to cause problems.
Relapse Stage Goal—Client learns from short-term success and reengages in the change process.	· Remind the client that it is common to "recycle." · Reframe from "failure" to "success for a while." · Focus on lessons learned and help the client to reengage in the change process.

Source: Modified from Zimmerman, G. L., Olsen, C. G., & Bosworth, M. F. (2000). A 'stages of change' approach to helping patients change behavior. *American Family Physician, 61,* p. 1412.)

Consciousness Raising

During the contemplation stage of behavior change, consciousness raising occurs as the client seeks information. The nurse can share potential resources and can help explain and interpret conflicting or unclear information. During this phase it is important to clarify the client's incentives and barriers to change, assess the knowledge and interest of family members, and can encourage the client to talk with others who have successfully made similar changes.

Self- and Environmental Reevaluation

The client will begin to engage in self- and environmental reevaluation while moving toward the preparation and action stages of change. Issues clients may consider include how the current problem behavior (or lack of positive behavior) affects the physical and social environment, and personal standards and values. Other questions clients might ask are: Will I like myself better as a (thinner, nonsmoking, less-stressed) individual? Is my environment supportive of the proposed changes? Do I believe that I am able to make and continue the changes needed? It is important for clients to face these questions because change will only occur when it is compatible with the client's self-concept.

Self- and Social Liberation

A strategy that can assist with self- and social liberation is cognitive restructuring. "Cognitive restructuring focuses on client's thinking, imagery, and attitudes toward the self and self-competencies as they affect the change process" (Pender, 1996, p. 171). The nurse can help clarify the messages clients tell themselves about their health and health-related behaviors. For example, certain beliefs or thoughts may be irrational or unfounded when compared with reality. Positive affirmations and imagery, repeated several times a day, can help clients think positively and make desired lifestyle changes.

Helping Relationships

Helping relationships with family members, friends, colleagues, or health-care professionals, are critical for moving the client through the preparation, action, and maintenance stages of change. A self-help or support group can provide valuable support, modeling, and reinforcement of the desired behavior.

Stimulus Control

Stimulus control emphasizes activities that precede the desired behavior, which can be helpful during the action and maintenance stages of change. The activities must be personally relevant to the client, and might include a postcard remainder for mammography screening, a personal call from the nurse to encourage continued exercise, or a scheduled group meeting to practice relaxation. To promote the development of a desirable behavior it may be helpful for the client to practice the behavior daily at the same time and in the same setting or context. For example, suggesting that the client exercise in the same place, early each morning before beginning other activities.

Counterconditioning

Counterconditioning is used to break an undesirable association between a stimulus and a response. This intervention can be useful during the later part of the action stage and during the maintenance stage. Undesirable associations can result from a negative emotional response to the desired behavior. For example, many clients indicate that exercise can become boring. In this situation the nurse can suggest alternatives, such as varied routine, walking outside when the weather permits, and exercising with a partner to counteract boredom.

Reinforcement Management

Reinforcement management is an effective strategy, especially during the preparation and action stages of change. "It is based on the premise that all behaviors are determined by their consequences. If positive consequences occur, the probability is high that the behavior will occur again. If negative consequences occur, the probability is low for the behavior's being repeated" (Pender, 1996, p. 172). Immediate reinforcement of the desired behavior is important, especially in the early phases of change. Personalized attention and positive verbal feedback are helpful. Eventually, a desirable consequence of the behavior can become an intrinsic reward. For example, a weekly scale reading indicating weight loss can be enough of a reward for the client to continue losing weight.

The object of these strategies is to decrease the barriers to and increase the incentives for behavior change. Barriers to change include a lack of control, knowledge, skills, facilities (e.g., a place to exercise), materials, clear goals, social support, time, and motivation. According to Leddy (1997), incentives to change behavior include an expectation of benefit; sense of personal responsibility; enjoyment of the activity; previous experience; guilt for not changing behavior; and support from family, peers, or professionals. Appropriate strategies to promote behavior change should encourage incentives and reduce barriers, and be based on an individualized assessment by the nurse in a collaborative relationship with the client.

Motivational Interviewing

Another intervention technique to encourage behavior change is motivational interviewing (MI). This style of relating focuses on increasing client readiness for change in behavior. Motivational interviewing has been defined as "a directive, client-centered counseling style for eliciting behavior change by helping clients to explore and resolve ambivalence" (Rollnick & Miller, 1995, p. 326). MI comprises two equally important phases: Phase I—building a therapeutic rapport and commitment with the client, and Phase II—facilitating the client's movement through decisional analysis and behavior change.

Based on the assumption that the motivation to change begins with the client (is not externally imposed), MI relies upon identifying and mobilizing the client's intrinsic values and goals to stimulate behavior change. Direct persuasion does not seem to be an effective method for helping clients resolve uncertainty about behavior change. Thus, the nurse's goals for this approach are to help clients express their ambivalence, clarify and resolve the impasse, and guide them toward an acceptable resolution that triggers a change in behavior. "The art of motivational interviewing is therefore a dance between two individuals suspending judgment and avoiding a confrontational style thereby minimizing defensive reactions by the patient" (Shinitzky, & Kub, 2001, p. 181). Specific behaviors that are characteristics of a motivational interviewing style include:

- Relating in a partnership relationship with the client rather than taking expert/recipient roles.
- Being quiet and eliciting the client's thoughts and feelings rather than using a persuasive, aggressive, or confrontational style.
- Developing discrepancies between the client's present behavior and valued goals, through discussion.
- Using reflective listening to understand the client's frame of reference.
- Expressing empathy, acceptance, and affirmation toward the client.
- Eliciting and selectively reinforcing the client's motivational statements acknowledging the problem, and the desire, intention, and ability to change.
- Monitoring the client's degree of readiness to change.
- Supporting self-efficacy.
- Affirming the client's freedom of choice and self-direction.
- Providing meaningful personal feedback.

Principles of motivational interviewing include: (Duran, 2003):

1. *Building rapport with a therapeutic interviewing style*—address the client by the appropriate title and last name; introduce self by professional title and name; sit closely at eye level; speak without hurriedness; convey interest and caring; use skills such as open-ended questions and reflective listening; elicit immediate problems or concerns that the client may have before moving on to a discussion of behavior change.
2. *Using strategies for minimizing resistance*—affirm the client's choices and control; avoid telling the client what to do couched in the form of giving advice; avoid imposing an agenda on the client.
3. *Exploring ambivalence*—help the client to see discrepancies between personal goals and the behavior in question. Yield to client-generated decisions about why and how to proceed with change.

Further emphasizing the need for strategies such as MI, is the fact that the average health-care provider interrupts a client's disclosures after 18 seconds. And research shows that 30% to 60% of medical information discussed in an encounter is forgotten (Shinitzky & Kub, 2001).

It has been found that 45 to 120 minutes and several days of training are needed to provide the skills necessary for effective motivational interviewing (Goldstein et al., 1998). A menu of strategies for exploring concerns and options for change with clients follows, with the least threatening strategies listed first. It is best to start with the strategies at the beginning of the list for clients less ready to change.

1. Ask about (target behavior) in detail, "Tell me about your (smoking)."
2. Ask about a typical day, "Describe your diet over the course of a typical day."
3. Ask about lifestyle and stresses, "What kind of stress are you under?"
4. Ask about health status, then the target behavior; a discussion about health concerns can lead to an open question, "I wonder where you feel your typical diet fits in?"
5. Ask first about the good aspects of the behavior, then the less good, "What are the good things about your smoking? What are the not-so-good aspects?" While the

goal is to explore concerns, it is important to recognize that less positive aspects are not necessarily concerns. However, the interviewer can use this discussion to generate questions, "I wonder, how much does (the less positive aspect) bother you?"

6. Provide information and ask, "What do you think?"
7. Ask about concerns directly but only if the client appears ready and willing to talk, "What concerns do you have about your diabetes?"
8. Ask about the next step, "I wonder where this leaves you now?"

Another approach has been used by the Mayo Clinic College of Medicine to teach motivational interviewing skills to first-year medical students. The course consists of five 2-hour sessions. The mnemonics FRAMES (feedback, responsibility, advice, menu, empathy, and self-efficacy) and OARES (open-ended questions, affirm, reflective listening, elicit self-motivational statements, and summarize) are used to illustrate the philosophy and principles of motivational interviewing. The course used both lecture and experiential teaching strategies. After participating in the course, 77% of the students expressed confidence in their understanding of MI, compared with just 2% before the course (Poirier, Clark, Cerhan, Pruthi, Geda, and Dale, 2004).

The Brief Negotiation Model

A brief clinical intervention (20% classroom and 80% observational) can produce better outcomes than simple advice. The brief negotiation model training program for healthcare professionals consists of 4 or 6 hours, or 1 to 2 days. A central tenet of the model is that only clients can change themselves. This shifts the balance of power in the traditionally defined nurse-client relationship, where the nurse tells the client what to do and how to do it, and assumes that the client will do it (Runkle, Osterholm, Hoban, McAdam, and Tull, 2000).

Given this change in philosophy, the program is designed to:

- Expose health professionals to a recommended model of behavior change counseling.
- Increase the satisfaction and confidence of health professionals in counseling for behavior change.
- Increase the likelihood of improved client health outcomes.

The training program is derived from the following related principles:

1. *Stages of change*—nurses need to match their responses appropriately to the client's stage of readiness for change.
2. *Reactance theory*—if clients are told what to do, many will do the opposite (resistance). Thus, lecturing and preaching are usually counterproductive.
3. *Change talk*—beliefs are more influenced by what clients say than by what others say to them. Nurses should invite clients to discuss their motivations and desires for change.
4. *Confidence matters*—confidence in the ability to change is a predictor of change, persistence, success, and actual health status.

The training program proceeds through several steps. The first step involves setting the stage by establishing rapport, defining the time available for the visit, explicitly asking the client's permission to discuss the behavior issue, listening reflectively, and negotiating the agenda for the visit. The second step entails exchanging information, and emphasizes the importance of the communication style. Suggestions for the nurse include demonstrating empathy, conveying a collaborative nonjudgmental attitude, communicating clearly and succinctly, presenting the facts and providing education, expressing concern, and eliciting the client's response to information. The third step is assessing the client's readiness to change. A good way to assess readiness is by having the client choose a number on a scale of 0 to 10 where "0" is not ready and "10" is very ready. With this insight the nurse can acknowledge and explore the client's choice, and respond based on the readiness for change. The fourth step provides ways to close the visit, such as summarizing what the client said, expressing confidence in the client's ability to make the change, and confirming the next steps toward change.

Patient-Centered Counseling Model

The Patient-Centered Counseling model (Rosal, Ebbeling, Lofgren, Ockene, Ockene, and Hebert, 2001) facilitates change and long-term maintenance in dietary behavior by assessing client needs and then tailoring an intervention to the client's stage in the process of change. In this model, the nurse's objectives are to increase the client's awareness of risks resulting from the current behavior; provide information; increase the client's confidence in the ability to make changes, and enhance skills needed for long-term maintenance of the behavior change. The steps in the model include a complete behavioral *assessment*, personalized *advisement* based on the client's health concerns and stated reasons for wanting to change behavior, *assistance* in change based on stage of readiness for change, goal setting, reassessment of self-efficacy, a behavioral contract, and *arrangement for follow-up* to prevent relapse and promote maintenance of the behavior change.

Relapse Prevention

Rothman (2000) argues that different mechanisms drive the initiation and maintenance of behavior change. Decisions regarding behavior initiation are believed to depend on favorable expectations regarding future outcomes, whereas decisions regarding maintenance of behavior are believed to depend on perceived satisfaction with the outcomes. Initiation of behavior is viewed as approach-based, where the progress toward goals is indicated by a decrease in the difference between a current state and a desired state (e.g., maintaining a low-fat diet in order to increase energy). In contrast, behavioral maintenance is conceptualized as avoidance-based, where progress is indicated by a sustained difference between a current state and an undesired state (e.g., maintaining a low-fat diet in order to avoid cardiovascular disease). This theory implies that specific strategies need to be devised to promote maintenance of behavior change (e.g., see examples of processes of change discussed previously), and that these will differ from strategies used to promote initiation of behavior change.

"Relapse refers to a breakdown or failure in a person's attempt to change or modify a particular habit pattern, such as stopping 'bad habits' or developing new, optimal health behaviors" (Marlatt & George, 1998, p. 33). Relapse during any treatment program is often viewed as a failure by both the client and nurse. When significant time and energy have been invested in promoting change, clients who fail are often labeled "noncompliant" or "unmotivated" (Zimmerman, Olsen, and Bosworth, 2000).

In one analysis, the highest risk categories for relapse were negative emotional states (35%), interpersonal conflict (16%), and social pressure (20%). If clients can cope effectively with guilt, conflict, and self-blame resulting from a lapse, the probability of relapse decreases significantly.

Relapse prevention (RP) combines behavioral skill training procedures, cognitive therapy, and lifestyle rebalancing. RP can be applied either as a maintenance strategy to prevent relapse or as a more general approach to lifestyle change. In the RP approach, relapse is viewed as a transitional process, a fork in the road, or a series of events that may or may not be followed by a return to the behavior's pretreatment level. The RP approach assumes that providing the client with the necessary skills and cognitive strategies can prevent a single lapse from snowballing into a total relapse (Marlatt & George, 1998).

Specific and global RP strategies include skill training, cognitive reframing to emphasize positive aspects of behavior change, and lifestyle rebalancing (Marlatt & George, 1998). It is important for clients to recognize high-risk situations that may precipitate or trigger a relapse, such as socializing with other smokers when the client is trying to stop smoking. Sometimes clients experience a sense of deprivation with a behavior change. To reduce these feelings the nurse can use remedial coping skill rehearsal in real-life situations, write an explicit therapeutic contract with the client, and use therapeutic dialogue to restore equilibrium between "shoulds" and "wants."

The implication is that success in maintaining long-term behavior change requires broad-spectrum approaches at all levels. However, very little is known about the mechanisms responsible for the most effective maintenance strategies, such as extended contact with a support person, telephone support, or supplying appropriate foods in diet and weight loss programs. Brief counseling sessions (lasting 5 to 15 minutes) have been just as effective as longer visits in reducing relapse. But most existing maintenance interventions are not effective, and "even the most promising interventions are limited in impact and poorly understood" (Orleans, 2000, p. 82). Theory-based intervention research to reduce relapse is badly needed.

Health Behavior Change Programs on the Internet

Thirty-seven Web sites for health behavior change or disease prevention and management were evaluated. "The strength of these 37 programs included: rationales provided for assessments; privacy and confidentiality protections; some form of feedback provided; and some form of interactivity. The weaknesses included: few were theory driven; few had individualized tailoring; few had empirically based tailoring; and few were evidence-based or reported subsequent plans for evaluation" (Evers, Prochaska, Prochaska, Driskell, Cummins, and Velicer, 2003, p. 63).

It has also been found that mediated health campaigns have only small measurable effects in the short-term. A meta-analysis (Snyder, Hamilton, Mitchell, Kiwanuka-Tondo, Fleming-Milici, and Proctor, 2004) showed that campaign effect sizes were very low (e.g., r=.15 for seat belt use, r=.13 for oral health, r=.09 for alcohol use reduction, r=.05 for heart disease prevention, r=.05 for smoking, r=.04 for mammography and cervical cancer screening, and r=.04 for sexual behaviors).

Suggestions for Health Behavior Change Interventions

Given that health behavior change is difficult for most individuals, some of the following suggestions may be helpful (Westberg & Jason, 1996). It is important for clients to:

- Endorse the need for change.
- Have "ownership" of the need for change.
- Feel that there is more to gain than to lose.
- Develop an enhanced sense of self-worth.
- Identify realistic goals and workable plans.
- Seek gradual change rather than a "quick fix."
- Have patience.
- Address starting new behaviors instead of just focusing on behaviors that should be stopped.
- Practice new behaviors.
- Seek the support of family, friends, colleagues, or health professionals.
- Gain positive reinforcement for the desired behavior.
- Have a strategy for monitoring progress and making needed changes.
- Seek constructive, personalized feedback to strengthen motivation for change.
- Have a mechanism of follow-up to reduce relapse.

Many interventions have focused on the initiation of behavior change at the level of individual illness and personal frailties. However, broad spectrum approaches are needed with interventions aimed at social and environmental policy, as well as practices influencing individual and group health. McKinlay (1995) uses a river metaphor to discuss "upstream" elements (public policy and environmental interventions), "midstream" elements (organizational channels such as schools, worksites, clinics and communities, and natural environments), and "downstream" elements (individuals at risk). The metaphor suggests that it doesn't make sense to keep rescuing drowning "downstream" individuals from the river without dealing with the "upstream" forces pushing them into the water. Success in maintaining long-term behavior change requires broad-spectrum interpersonal, community, environmental, and health-care system approaches as well as individual interventions.

References

Clark, N. M., & Becker, M. H. (1998). Theoretical models and strategies for improving adherence and disease management. In S. A. Schumaker, E. B. Schron, J. K. Oksene, & W. L. McBee (Eds.), *The handbook of human behavior change* (2nd ed., pp. 5–32). New York: Springer.

DiClemente, C. C., Marinilli, A. S., Singh, M., & Bellino, L. E. (2001). The role of feedback in the process of health behavior change. *American Journal of Health Behavior, 25,* 217–227.

Duran, L. S. (2003). Motivating health: Strategies for the nurse practitioner. *Journal of the American Academy of Nurse Practitioners, 15,* 200–205.

Evers, K. E., Prochaska, J. M., Prochaska, J. O., Driskell, M., Cummins, C. O., & Velicer, W. F. (2003). Strengths and weaknesses of health behavior change programs on the internet. *Journal of Health Psychology, 8,* 63–70.

Goldstein, M. G., DePue, J., Kazura, A., & Niaura, R. (1998). Models for provider-patient interaction: Applications to health behavior change. In S. A. Schumaker, E. B. Schron, J. K. Ockene, & W. L. McBee (Eds.), *The handbook of health behavior change* (2nd ed.). New York: Springer.

Leddy, S. K. (1997). Incentives and barriers to exercise in women with a history of breast cancer. *Oncology Nursing Forum, 24,* 885–890.

Marlatt, G. A., & George, W. H. (1998). Relapse prevention and the maintenance of optimal health. In S. A. Schumaker, E. B. Schron, J. K. Ocktene, & W. L. McBee. *The handbook of health behavior change* (2nd ed.). New York: Springer.

McKinlay, J. B. (1995). The promotion of health through planned sociopolitical change. Challenges for research and policy. *Social Science and Medicine, 36,* 109–117.

Miller, W. R., & Rollnick, S. (1991). *Motivational interviewing: Preparing people to change addictive behavior.* New York: Guilford.

Orleans, C. T. (2000). Promoting the maintenance of health behavior change: Recommendations for the next generation of research and practice. *Health Psychology, 19*(Suppl.), 76–83.

Pender, N. J. (1996). *Health promotion in nursing practice* (3rd ed.). Stamford, CT: Appleton & Lange.

Peterson, J., Atwood, J. R., & Yates, B. (2002). Key elements for church-based health promotion programs: Outcome-based literature review. *Public Health Nursing, 19,* 401–411.

Poirier, M. K., Clark, M. M., Cerhan, J. H., Pruthi, S., Geda, Y. E., & Dale, L. C. (2004). Teaching motivational interviewing to first-year medical students to improve counseling skills in health behavior change. *Mayo Clinical Proceedings, 79,* 327–331.

Prochaska, J. O., Velicer, W. F., Rossi, J. S., Goldstein, M. G., Marcus, B., Rakowski, W., Fiore, C., et al. (1994). Stages of change and decisional balance for 12 problem behaviors. *Health Psychology, 13,* 39–46.

Rollnick, S., Mason, P., & Butler, C. (1999). *Health behavior change: A guide for practitioners.* Edinburgh: Churchill Livingstone.

Rollnick, S., & Miller, W. R. (1995). What is motivational interviewing? *Behavioral and Cognitive Psychotherapy, 23,* 325–334.

Rosal, M. C., Ebbeling, C. B., Lofgren, I., Ockene, J., Ockene, I. S., & Hebert, J. R. (2001). Facilitating dietary change: The patient-centered counseling model. *Journal of the American Dietetic Association, 101,* 332–338, 341.

Rothman, A. J. (2000). Toward a theory-based analysis of behavioral maintenance. *Health Psychology, 19,* 64–69.

Runkle, C., Osterholm, A., Hoban, R., McAdam, E., & Tull, R. (2000). Brief negotiation program for promoting behavior change: The Kaiser Permanente approach to continuing professional development. *Education for Health, 13,* 377–386.

Shinitzky, H. E., & Kub, J. (2001). The art of motivating behavior change: The use of motivational interviewing to promote health. *Public Health Nursing, 18,* 178–185.

Snyder, L. B., Hamilton, M. A., Mitchell, E. W., Kiwanuka-Tondo, J., Fleming-Milici, F., & Proctor, D. (2004). A meta-analysis of the effect of mediated health communication campaigns on behavior change in the United States. *Journal of Health Communication, 9,* 71–96.

Sue, D. W. (2002). Cultural competence in behavior health care. In J. C. Chung (Ed.), *The human behavioral change imperative: Theory, education, and practice in diverse populations* (pp. 41–50). New York: Kluwer Academic/Plenum.

Walsh, J. M., & McPhee, S. J. (1992) A systems model of clinical preventive care: An analysis of factors influencing patient and physician. *Health Education Quarterly, 19,* 157–175.

Westberg, J., & Jason, H. (1996). Fostering healthy behavior: The process. In S. H. Woolf, S. Jonas,

& R. S. Lawrence (Eds.), *Health promotion and disease prevention in clinical practice* (pp. 145–162). Baltimore: Williams & Wilkins.

Zimmerman, G. L., Olsen, C. G., & Bosworth, M. F. (2000). A 'stages of change' approach to helping patients change behavior. *American Family Physician, 61,* 1409–1416.

CHAPTER 15

A Summary of Nursing Interventions

Concepts
Nurse-Client Relationship
Communication/Support
Motivation
Teaching
Reframing
Stress Reduction

Helpful Lists
Principles for Strengths-Based Nursing
   Practice, pg. 192

Strengthening Client-Nurse
   Relationships, pg. 193
Relatedness Social Activities, pg. 193
False Assumptions, pg. 194
Strategies to Improve Nurse-Client
   Communication, pgs. 194–195
Countering Techniques, pg. 197
Reframing Techniques, pg. 197
Additional Intervention Strategies,
   pgs. 198–199
Intervention Do's and Don'ts,
   pgs. 199–200

Thought Questions

1. What changes do you plan to implement in the way you practice nursing after reading this book?
2. How would you summarize the elements of a strengths approach to nursing practice?
3. How can you integrate individual health behavior change strategies into institutional or community-based nursing practice? Can you identify at least ten strategies that you could implement immediately?
4. How can you integrate strength-based interventions into nursing practice? Can you identify at least five strategies that you could implement immediately?

Chapter Synopsis

This chapter reviews intervention strategies that have been discussed in previous chapters. It should be remembered that the Healthiness Theory is a unitary theory, meaning that all the concepts are inseparable in reality. Therefore, the nurse needs to integrate the strategies from individual chapters into a cohesive whole for practice. This chapter is designed to help with that process, through sections on the nurse-client relationship, communications/support, motivation, teaching, reframing, and stress reduction.

CHANGING FOCUS

Traditional professional health care is based on the belief that something about the client is "broken" and needs to be "fixed." Within most health-related professions, including nursing, it is assumed that the expertise of the professional and the mastering of theories, practice skills, and experience will make the difference in the client's life. However, health-care techniques or interventions are responsible for only about 15% of the outcome (Blundo, 2001). Ultimately, most of the change that occurs is a result of what the client brings to the process. The client's strengths, resilience, and social supports are responsible for what is going to change and how it changes. Thus, nurses need to understand how clients make changes and know how to support the change process in the most productive way. This implies a shift from focusing on the problems and deficits as defined by the nurse, to focusing on client possibilities and strengths.

The strengths perspective requires a significant change in how nurses think about clients and their families, how they think about themselves as professionals, the nature of the knowledge base for practice, and the process of nursing practice. What is needed is an egalitarian, collaborative working relationship in a strengths/solution-based practice (Blundo, 2001). By intentionally intervening, the nurse can help clients change perspective on a problem, give up unattainable goals, and plan a course of action; elicit and use information about available resources; anticipate future problems, self-regulate behavior, and persevere rather than giving up (Aspinwall & Staudinger, 2003; Caprara & Cervone, 2003). In order to promote these outcomes, the nurse must understand the developmental, material, and social contexts that support or hinder human strengths.

GENERAL PRINCIPLES FOR STRENGTHS-BASED NURSING PRACTICE

1. Negotiate desired approaches and outcomes with clients rather than forcing them to pursue specific outcomes selected by the nurse.
2. Focus money and time on educating clients about using their strengths and finding ways to build on them, rather than trying to plug "skill gaps."
3. Maximize client functioning with problems instead of trying to move them to a state of functioning without problems.
4. Focus on client strengths and assets *along with* deficits and problems, in order to design interventions *both* to increase assets and decrease problems (Graybeat, 2001; Kivnick & Murray, 2001).

THE NURSE-CLIENT RELATIONSHIP

It has been stated that a therapeutic relationship accounts for 30% of the improvement in clients' lives (in addition to the effect of care-based interventions) (Keyes & Lopez, 2002). How can a nurse best use each interaction in a therapeutic way in a limited time? The recommendations that follow should help nurses develop and strengthen client-nurse relationships:

1. Recognize the importance of being rather than doing, within a context of exchange and sharing.
2. Validate the client's experiences while encouraging hope.
3. Acknowledge reciprocity, equity, and the give and take of relationships over time.
4. Identify shared commonalities that validate the client through personal presence, open communication, an unconditional relationship, respect, trust, partnership, and silence.
5. Balance interdependence and interrelatedness. Specifically, enhance the client's sense of control through modeling behavior, encouraging participation in treatment decisions, using positive self-talk, and identifying controllable and uncontrollable events in the client's life (Lazarus & Folkman, 1984).
6. Help clients help themselves by emphasizing self-reliance, autonomy, and empowerment.
7. Communicate trust, praise positive behavior, encourage choice, and affirm the client's perspective.
8. Implement models of service delivery that "emphasize self-reliance and autonomy, promote supportive environments, enhance access to user-friendly healthcare information, and address the needs of informal support networks" (Forbes, 2001, p. 32).
9. Build rapport with a therapeutic interviewing style. Address the client by appropriate title and last name; introduce self by professional title and name; sit closely at eye level; speak without hurriedness; convey interest and caring; use skills such as open-ended questions and reflective listening; and elicit the client's immediate problems or concerns.
10. Use strategies to minimize resistance. Affirm the client's choices and control; avoid telling the client what to do couched in the form of giving advice; and avoid imposing an agenda on the client.

The human tendency to form strong, stable interpersonal bonds is referred to as the "need to belong." It is important for nurses to identify their own needs for relatedness and feeling close and connected to significant others outside the work environment, without transferring that need inappropriately to client relationships (Reis, Sheldon, Gable, Roscoe, and Ryan, 2000). Reis and colleagues (2000) have identified types of social activity that contribute to a sense of relatedness:

1. Communicating about personally relevant matters within a context of shared commonalities
2. Participating in shared activities
3. Spending informal social time with a group of friends
4. Feeling understood and appreciated
5. Participating in pleasant or otherwise enjoyable activities
6. Avoiding arguments and conflict that create distance and feelings of disengagement with significant others
7. Avoiding self-conscious or insecure feelings that direct attention toward the self and away from others

Communication skills are very important when establishing and maintaining a therapeutic nurse-client relationship. The following section presents strategies to enhance nurse-client communication and support.

COMMUNICATION/SUPPORT

Communication is improved when the nurse focuses on the treatment plan, has a congenial demeanor, and uses reassuring communication (Clark & Becker, 1998). Other strategies include being attentive to the client; asking about the client's underlying concerns; addressing the immediate concerns of the family; engaging the client in conversation via open-ended questions, using simple language and analogies to teach important concepts; tailoring the therapeutic regimen when needed; using appropriate nonverbal encouragement and verbal praise for successes; constructing reassuring messages to alleviate fears; eliciting the client's immediate objective and reaching an agreement with the client and the family on a short-term goal; and reviewing the long-term plan for the client's treatment so the client knows what to expect.

It is not uncommon to make assumptions about clients, and it is important to be aware of false assumptions that the nurse may hold such as (Rollnick, Mason, and Butler, 1999, pp. 34–35):

1. This client OUGHT to change. Fact: Change depends on the client and their perceived need for change, not whether the nurse thinks it is important.
2. This client WANTS to change. Fact: Clients often have conflicting motives and feelings about making a change.
3. The client's health is the prime motivating factor. Fact: There may be other factors that provide greater motivation for change. The nurse can help clients discern their motives and act on them effectively. Health doesn't have to be the prime motivator for a client to make a healthy change.
4. If the client does not decide to change, the consultation has failed. Fact: Deciding to change is a process, not an event, and it takes time.
5. Clients are either motivated to change, or not. Fact: The motivation to do something is not an all or nothing phenomenon; it is a matter of degree.
6. Now is the right time to consider change. Fact: But it might not be the best time for the client.
7. A tough approach is always best. Fact: Most clients do not respond well to authoritative communication, which can result in the client resisting change.
8. The nurse is the expert and the client must follow the advice given. Fact: Telling the client what to do does not encourage behavior change. When clients are equal partners in their care they are more willing to take responsibility for change.

Specific strategies to improve nurse-client communication include:

1. Relating in a partnership relationship in contrast to taking expert/recipient roles.
2. Listening and being nonjudgmental about the client's concerns and issues.
3. Having direct and respectful (assertive) communication of needs and desires

so others can understand and decide whether or not they can accommodate requests.

4. Practicing active listening to understand and interpret accurately another individual's message.
5. Being present while probing for a deeper understanding and paraphrasing back what was heard (Fletcher, 2004).
6. Being quiet and eliciting rather than using a persuasive, aggressive, or confrontational style.
7. Using reflective listening to understand the client's frame of reference.
8. Expressing empathy, acceptance, and affirmation.
9. Eliciting and selectively reinforcing the client's motivational statements regarding their recognition of problems, and the desire, intention, and ability to change.
10. Monitoring the client's degree of readiness for new behaviors.
11. Supporting self-efficacy.
12. Affirming the client's freedom of choice and self-direction.
13. Providing meaningful personal feedback and eliciting the client's response.
14. Communicating clearly and succinctly.
15. Presenting the facts and providing information and education.

One element of supportive communication includes helping relationships. Specific social support interventions may include: cognitive therapy strategies, such as correcting distorted thinking related to a client's distressed mood (gather information); and training in social skills (initiate conversation, facilitate dialogue, foster the ability to talk about interests, increase self-disclosure, encourage the expression of emotion; and use reflective journaling). Pierce and colleagues (1996) found that the following considerations were important for developing connectedness: physical presence; expressions of concern; calm acceptance; expression of optimism; provision of useful information or advice; expression of special understanding because of similar experience; provision of technically competent care; and being pleasant and kind.

However, "studies designed to increase perceived social support have not provided strong evidence that social support can be improved very easily" (Lakey & Lutz, 1996, p. 446). The nurse can only provide limited social support for the client, and should encourage the client's ability to garner support from others.

MOTIVATION

Personal control is one of the most important factors determining whether or not an individual will be open to change (Peterson & Stunkard, 1989). As clients engage in self- and environmental reevaluation, they may consider how an increase in positive attitudes and behavior can affect the physical and social environment, and personal standards and values. Questions that the client might ask include: Will I like myself better as a (thinner, nonsmoking, less-stressed) individual? Is my environment supportive of the proposed changes? Do I believe that I am able to make and continue the changes needed? Changes will only occur when they fit with an individual's self-concept.

The complexity that can make change seem overwhelming to the client can be modified by prioritizing the regimen, by breaking the treatment plan into less complex stages that can be implemented sequentially; and by minimizing both inconvenience and forgetfulness by tailoring the regimen schedule to the client's regular activities. As noted earlier, a client's behavior change skills deteriorate over time when they are not used. Clients must know how to determine if the regimen is working and be able to identify signs of problems, should they occur (Clark & Becker, 1998). The nurse can help the client explore feelings of ambivalence, and should yield to client-generated decisions about why and how to proceed with change. Teaching strategies can help clients to see the discrepancy between their personal goals and behavior.

TEACHING

Consciousness raising occurs as the client seeks information. The nurse can share potential resources and can help explain and interpret conflicting or unclear information. During this phase the nurse can clarify the client's incentives and barriers to change, and assess the knowledge and interest of family members. The nurse can also encourage the client to talk with others who successfully made similar changes.

When planning for an information sharing session, the nurse should consider the following characteristics of recall. Recall varies according to the timing of messages (material presented in the first third of the discussion is best remembered). Selective recall indicates that clients usually recall the diagnosis better than the therapy recommendations. Recall can be enhanced through labeling and categorizing messages (simple reorganization of a list of 15 medical statements into labeled categories enhanced recall by 50%), and recall through recognition (well-organized messages repeated several times in a simple leaflet significantly improved adherence to a weight-loss plan) (Clark & Becker, 1998).

If clients are told what to do in an authoritative manner, they will often resist and do the opposite. By implication, lecturing and preaching are counterproductive. Further, beliefs are influenced more by what a client says than by what others say to them. The client's confidence in the ability to change is a predictor of change, persistence, success, and perceptions of health.

REFRAMING

"Cognitive restructuring focuses on client's thinking, imagery, and attitudes toward the self and self-competencies as they affect the change process" (Pender, 1996, p. 171). Reframing promotes flexible thought and resiliency by transforming negative thinking into positive thinking (Keyes & Lopez, 2002). What may appear to be insurmountable obstacles can be reframed as challenges. Positive reappraisal involves focusing on the good in present and past events. Techniques for promoting emotional expression and insight include mind monitoring and thought changing, self-talk, relaxation techniques, meditation, and various imaging methods. The emphasis is on changing the client's state of mind rather than on manipulating external circumstances.

Another strategy is called countering, or using an alternative to negative thinking. Countering techniques can include:

- Decreasing subjective distress by visualizing a pleasant scene or using relaxation techniques
- Using thought-stopping techniques, such as clapping hands or snapping a rubber band at the wrist
- Neutralizing thinking by getting rid of distractions, distorted thoughts, and other preoccupations
- Visualizing a positive outcome (Davidhizar & Shearer, 1996)

Other helpful strategies the nurse can use to promote positive thinking and enhance the client's confidence include, (1) listening for recurrent negative themes and helping the client change them, (2) modeling positive thinking, and (3) encouraging the client to read books and attend workshops that may be helpful. As clients recognize the beginning signs of positive thinking, giving themselves positive feedback helps to reinforce positive thoughts and feelings (Davidhizar & Shearer, 1996). The nurse can help clarify the messages clients give themselves about their health and health-related behaviors. For example, certain beliefs or thoughts may be irrational or unfounded when compared with reality. Positive affirmations and imagery, repeated several times a day, can help clients think positively and make desired lifestyle changes.

The effects of reframing first occur with changes in positive and negative thoughts and in beliefs about self and outcomes (Lightsey, 1996). Suggestions to assist clients with reframing their thinking include:

1. Concentrating on helping clients to develop self-efficacy and outcome expectancies (or goals) at specific and general levels. The ultimate goal should be to help clients change schemata.
2. Using a variety of interventions to increase capability beliefs, including graded mastery experiences, verbal persuasion, vicarious learning, and an interpretation of the client's physiological/emotional state.
3. Integrating homework that involves graded but powerful mastery experiences in areas valued by the client.
4. Encouraging the expression of positive and negative emotions. Increased disclosure is associated with decreased sympathetic nervous system activity and increased immune system activity.
5. Helping the client increase positive thoughts/beliefs and decrease negative thoughts/beliefs. Strive for a lot more positive thinking relative to negative thinking.
6. Helping the client to develop active problem-solving skills.
7. Teaching a variety of proactive coping skills.
8. Using a variety of modalities to effect change in schemata. Use visual imagery, which is closely tied to stimulation of schemata.
9. Cultivating knowledge of the client's culture.
10. Paying attention to human commonalities across cultures.
11. Finding an outlet for expression of emotion.
12. Preparing clients to encounter negative thinking from others.

STRESS REDUCTION

Relaxation therapies (e.g., meditation, yoga, progressive muscle relaxation, biofeedback, and imagery using selected nature scenes) cultivate feelings of contentment. Relaxation therapies also provide practical skills for interacting with the external environment, developing more complex and resilient views of the self, improving immune functioning, and even extending life (Fredrickson, 2000).

Additional Intervention Strategies

1. Attributional probing—reveals faulty assumptions, distorted self-defeating attitudes, and unresolved existential conflicts.
2. Life review and play back—allows the client to reminisce.
3. Fast-forwarding—depicts likely scenarios that might result from a particular choice.
4. Magical thinking—transcends present thinking (if you were free to do whatever you want and money was not an issue, what would you like to do?).
5. Constructing a personal meaning profile—components might include religion, positive relationships, achievement, self-transcendence, self-acceptance, meaning and purpose, and self-realization.
6. Targeting and contracting—focuses on attainable goals. Have the client complete assignments or practice new skills.
7. Effective coping—means accepting life's realities and learning to reframe thinking to look for positive meanings in negative life events.
8. Overcoming the Achilles' heel—clients are often their own worst enemies. They may be self-destructive, or something may be holding them back from achieving their full potential.
9. Promoting belonging or social support (e.g., support groups, clubs, or drop-in programs).
10. Promoting capability and providing feedback about skill level (e.g., involvement in sports and recreation programs; volunteer and paid employment experiences).
11. Promoting self-awareness (e.g., self-discovery programs, involvement in values clarification exercises and workshops).
12. Providing instruction in the fundamental skills needed for belonging (e.g., programs that assist the client in developing proactive social skills).
13. Considering ways of stimulating the client's environment to bring about the desired goals.
14. Referring clients to pastoral staff and qualified counselors to assist with issues concerning spirituality, belonging, and vocational guidance.
15. Encouraging creative expression and personal style in the performance of everyday activities.
16. Focusing on goals, obstacles, alternative routes to goals, and determination in pursuit of goals (Michael, Taylor, and Cheavens, 2000).

17. Using language and examples, or employing visual aids and activities that fit clients' abilities to comprehend and express themselves.
18. Encouraging the client to maintain a daily diary to document self-monitoring and cognitive restructuring. The client can rate good and bad events, both internal and external, and discern their possible causes.
19. Helping the client identify and modify dysfunctional optimism that leads to suppressing beliefs, and identify beneficial alternative views.
20. Encouraging positive visualization to identify possible problems and ways of coping. This can include "storyboarding," which involves visualizing discrete scenes that lead to a desired outcome, and "invulnerability training" to promote good feelings about how a particular situation was handled.
21. Considering the use of the "silver lining" technique to try to find a positive benefit in a negative experience.
22. Considering the use of "pump priming," where clients attend to experiences relevant to a schema the client wants to encourage.
23. Having the client complete an "antiprocrastination sheet" to express how difficult or how rewarding it was to perform a task. This list can include the best, worst, and most likely outcome.
24. Encouraging relaxation, meditation, and stress-reduction skills to help in the management of negative affect (NA).
25. Facilitating problem-solving and task management strategies.

Some specific do's and don'ts for clients trying to achieve goals include the following suggestions (Lopez, Floyd, Ulven, and Snyder 2000):

DO

- Break a long-range goal into steps or subgoals.
- Begin to pursue a distant goal by concentrating on short-term goals.
- Practice planning different routes to goals and select the best one.
- Mentally practice the actions needed to accomplish the goal.
- Mentally rehearse scripts about how to react in the event of a blockage.
- When a goal is not reached, conclude that the strategy was unworkable, don't self-blame.
- If a new skill is necessary to reach the goal, learn it.
- Cultivate two-way friendships, be willing to give and receive advice.
- Be willing to ask for help in reaching a desired goal. Take "ownership" of the need for change.
- Feel that there is more to gain than to lose.
- Develop an enhanced sense of self-worth.
- Identify realistic goals and workable plans.
- Seek gradual change rather than a "quick fix."
- Have patience.
- Address starting new behaviors instead of just focusing on stopping negative behaviors.
- Practice new behaviors.
- Seek the support of family, friends, colleagues, or health professionals.

- Gain positive reinforcement for the desired behavior.
- Have a strategy for monitoring progress and making needed changes.
- Seek constructive, personalized feedback to strengthen the motivation for change.
- Have a mechanism of follow-up to reduce relapse.

DON'T

- Think big goals can be accomplished all at once.
- Be too hurried in producing routes to goals.
- Be rushed to select the best or first route to the goal.
- Overanalyze with the idea of finding one perfect route to the goal.
- Stop thinking about alternate strategies when one doesn't work.
- Self-blame when an initial strategy fails.
- Be caught off guard when one approach doesn't work.
- Get into friendships where there is praise for not coming up with solutions to problems (Westberg & Jason, 1996).

References

Aspinwall, L. G., & Studinger, U. M. (2003). A psychology of human strengths: Some central issues of an emerging field. *A psychology of personal strengths. Fundamental questions and future directions for a positive psychology* (pp. 9–22). Washington, DC: American Psychological Association.

Blundo, R. (2001). Learning strengths-based practice: Challenging our personal and professional frames. *Families in Society: The Journal of Contemporary Human Services, 82,* 296–304.

Caprara, G. V., & Cervone, D. (2003). A conception of personality for a psychology of human strengths: Personality as an agentic, self-regulating system. In L. G. Aspinwall & U. M. Studinger (Eds.), *A psychology of human strengths. Fundamental questions and future directions for a positive psychology* (pp. 61–74). Washington, DC: American Psychological Association.

Clark, N. M., & Becker, M. H. (1998). Theoretical models and strategies for improving adherence and disease management. In S. A. Schumaker, E. B. Schron, J. K. Oksene, & W. L. McBee (Eds.), *The handbook of human behavior change* (2nd ed., pp. 5–32). New York: Springer.

Davidhizar, R. E., & Shearer, R. (1996). Increasing self-confidence through self-talk. *Home Healthcare Nurse, 14,* 119–122.

Fletcher, S. K. (2004). Religion and life meaning: Differentiating between religious beliefs and religious community in constructing life meaning. *Journal of Aging Studies, 18,* 171–185.

Forbes, E. A. (2001). Enhancing mastery and sense of coherence: Important determinants of health in older adults. *Geriatric Nursing, 22,* 29–32.

Fredrickson, B. L. (2000). Cultivating positive emotions to optimize health and well-being. *Prevention and Treatment, 3,* 1–25.

Graybeat, C. (2001). Strengths-based social work assessment: Transforming the dominant paradigm. *Families in Society: The Journal of Contemporary Human Services, 82,* 233–242.

Keyes, C. L. M., & Lopez, S. J. (2002). Toward a science of mental health. In C. R. Snyder & S. J. Lopez (Eds.), *Handbook of positive psychology* (pp. 45–59). Oxford: Oxford University Press.

Kivnick, H. Q., & Murray, S. V, (2001). Life strengths interview guide: Assessing elder clients' strengths. *Journal of Gerontological Social Work, 34,* 7–31.

Lakey, B., & Lutz, C. J. (1996). Social support and preventive and therapeutic interventions. In G. R. Pierce, B. R. Sarason, & I. G. Sarason (Eds.), *Handbook of social support and the family* (pp. 435–465). New York: The Plenum Press.

Lazarus, R. S., & Folkman, S. (1984). *Stress, appraisal and coping.* New York: Springer.

Lightsey, O. R. (1996). What leads to wellness? The role of psychological resources in well-being. *The Counseling Psychologist, 24,* 589–735.

Lopez, S. J., Floyd, R. K., Ulvan, J. C., & Snyder, C. R. (2000). Hope therapy: Helping clients build a house of hope. In C. R. Snyder (Ed.), *Handbook of hope: Theory, measures and applications* (pp. 123–150). San Diego, CA: Academic Press.

Michael, S. T., Taylor, J. D., & Cheavens, J. (2000). Hope theory as applied to brief treatments: Problem-solving and solution-focused therapies. In C. R. Snyder (Ed.), *Handbook of hope: Theory, measures and applications* (pp. 151–166). San Diego, CA: Academic Press.

Pender, N. J. (1996). *Health promotion in nursing practice* (3rd ed.). Stamford, CT: Appleton & Lange.

Peterson, C., & Stunkard, A. J. (1989). Personal control and health promotion. *Social Science and Medicine, 28,* 819–828.

Pierce, G. R., Sarason, B. R., Sarason, I. G., Joseph, H. J., & Henderson, C. A. (1996). Conceptualizing and assessing social support in the context of the family. In G. R. Pierce, B. R. Sarason, & I. G. Sarason (Eds.), *Handbook of social support and the family* (pp. 3–23). New York: The Plenum Press.

Reis, H. T., Sheldon, K. M., Gable, S. L., Roscoe, J., & Ryan, R. M. (2000). Daily well-being: The role of autonomy, competence, and relatedness. *Personality and Social Psychology, 26,* 419–435.

Rollnick, S., Mason, P., & Butler, C. (1999). *Health behavior change: A guide for practitioners.* Edinburgh: Churchill Livingstone.

Westberg, J., & Jason, H. (1996). Fostering healthy behavior: The process. In S. H. Woolf, S. Jonas, & R. S. Lawrence (Eds.), *Health promotion and disease prevention in clinical practice* (pp. 145–162). Baltimore: Williams & Wilkins.

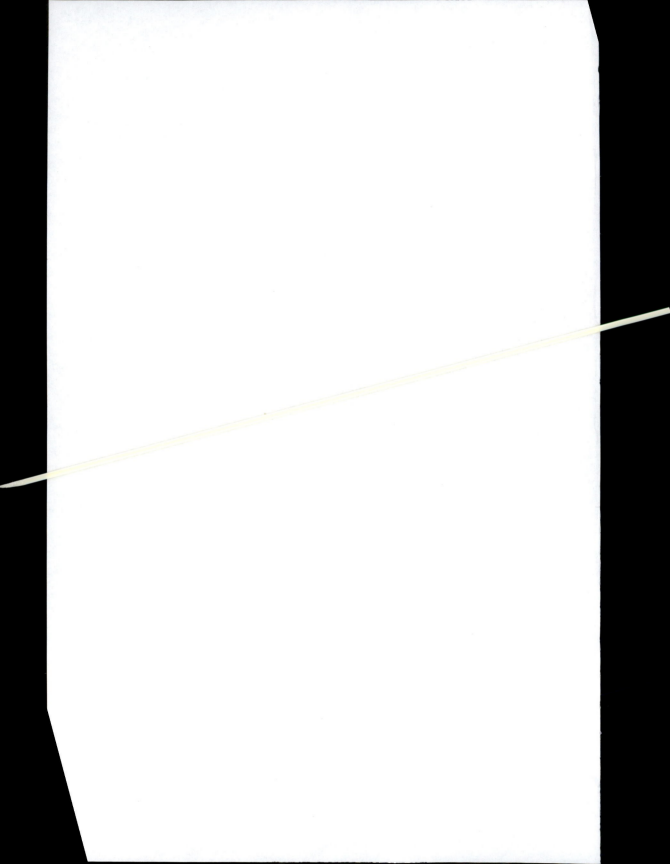

Health Promotion: Mobilizing Strengths to Enhance Health, Wellness, and Well-Being

INTRODUCTION OF CASE STUDIES

The intent of the following three brief case studies is to suggest differences between the current traditional model of "problem-oriented" nursing care, and the strengths approach to care. The separation of these approaches is an artificial strategy to differentiate between them for teaching purposes. But, in practice, the approaches should be integrated to provide comprehensive client care that is oriented toward well-being and quality of life. The ideal nursing interventions would include both approaches, and would strengthen all of the concepts as resources for health, provide choices (alternatives) rather than "telling," present challenges rather than threats, and would be based on a trusting, ongoing relationship exemplified by genuineness, mutuality, and nurse-client shared power.

CASE STUDY I

Pam Jones is a 53-year-old woman who has had full responsibility for the care of her 83-year-old mother, who has had Alzheimer's disease for the past 8 years. On a routine visit to the Geriatric Clinic you identify the following concerns by talking about her role as a caregiver.

1. Has not had a Pap test for 6 years, and has never had a mammogram.
2. Eats a high-starch, high-sugar diet, and is 25% above ideal body weight.
3. Complains of an overwhelming sense of fatigue, and is having increasing difficulty carrying out necessary daily activities.
4. Has no regular exercise program.
5. Complains of having a constant, dull headache and is occasionally unable to concentrate.
6. Has had no relief from caregiving responsibility.
7. Quit work 6 years ago to care for her mother full-time, and has limited social relationships.

continues

continued from previous page

Problem Approach	Strengths Approach
1. *Encourage Ms. Jones to arrange to have a mammogram and gyn exam.*	Encourage a mammogram and gyn exam.
2. *Tell Ms. Jones that her diet and weight put her at risk for diabetes and heart problems. Ask her if she would like to talk with a dietitian.*	Emphasize increasing energy, and feeling good while losing weight. Focus on improved *self-confidence, capacity*, and *capability*. For example, point out any negative thinking that may be blocking her belief in the ability to lose weight. This might help her feel more confident in making an appointment with a dietitian. Also, breaking the amount of weight she needs to lose into a weekly amount may help her feel more in control and more capable.
3.–4. *Encourage Ms. Jones to rest when she feels tired.*	An activity program, if it incorporates *challenge,* can increase *capacity.* The focus should be on improving her perception of having *choices* for activities and scheduling, For example, help Ms. Jones think about different options that might provide opportunities for rest.
5. *Suggest over-the-counter headaches remedies. Express sympathy for her difficult situation.*	Teach Ms. Jones proactive coping strategies to reduce stress. Help her to identify *meaning* in her life, and a few *goals* to reduce the feeling of being overwhelmed and increase her perception of *control.* For example, suggest that a religious advisor might be helpful in identifying meaning and purpose in her life.
6.–7. *Ask if her daughter can help out.*	Ms. Jones needs *connections* for social support and tangible assistance. Help her to identify Alzheimer's support groups. With her approval, set up a social worker consultation for possible respite resource *choices.*

CASE STUDY II

Carol Peters is a 32-year-old, unmarried secretary who has just delivered her first child, a girl she named Susan. Susan, was 7 pounds 12 ounces at birth, and was delivered vaginally, with only one dose of medication when Ms. Peters was 6 cm dilated. She wants to breast-feed. In caring for Ms. Peters throughout her labor and delivery you have identified the following concerns:

1. Financial concerns. She needs to work. But, who will care for Susan?
2. Knows little about how to care for a newborn baby.

3. Does not expect to maintain contact with the father of the baby.
4. Estranged from her mother and sister, who live nearby, since her pregnancy.
5. Is bleeding vaginally.
6. Gained 60 pounds with the pregnancy. She complains that she "looks terrible."

Problem Approach	Strengths Approach
1. *Arrange for a social work consult.*	A social worker will be most able to help identify possible financial resources. But, this needs to be a decision she makes (*goals, challenge,* and *capability*).
2. *Encourage Ms. Peters to attend the parenting class offered by the hospital.*	The class is fine, but not enough. The nurse could enhance *control* by teaching her (by demonstration and repeat demonstration): • How to put a diaper on the baby • How to bathe and position the baby for sleep • How to breast-feed the baby, including the importance of colostrum She needs to know when to call the doctor (e.g., jaundice). The social worker might be able to find a support parenting group in the community.
3—4. *Encourage relationships.*	Ms. Peters will need tangible and instrumental social support. This includes helping her to gain *self-confidence* to reach out to her family (will also provide *connections*). The social work consult can provide assistance and possible *choices.*
5. *Provide perineal care.*	Enhance her perception of *capability* by teaching her how to do her own perineal care. Also teach her about massaging her abdomen to reduce bleeding, relief of possible hemorrhoids, possible breast engorgement, and how to relieve "afterpains."
6. *Urge her to exercise and try to lose 3 pounds a week.*	She needs to eat a nutritious diet to maintain her *capacity* and provide breast milk for Susan. Provide *choices* of foods she might eat, and discuss conservation of her energy.

Ms. Peters is going to need informational and tangible support to raise Susan on her own. She should be referred for public health nursing visits for the short-term, and choices of community resources for the longer-term. Every effort should be made, with her agreement, for her to reconcile with her family.

CASE STUDY III

Sam Smith is a 60-year-old accountant who has been hospitalized for 10 days. He has been diagnosed with acute myelogenous leukemia (AML), and has just completed a 5-day

continues

continued from previous page

course of aggressive induction chemotherapy with cytarabine and daunorubicin. Sam has been married to Joyce, a registered nurse, for 35 years. They have three grown children, and five grandchildren. You have identified the following concerns:

1. Has neutropenia, thrombocytopenia, and anemia as a result of the chemotherapy.
2. Has lost 10 pounds in the past week from diarrhea, anorexia, and painful mouth sores. He has a low-grade fever.
3. Complains of profound fatigue with weakness, and disturbed sleep.
4. Has petechiae on his legs and a large bruise on his left arm.
5. Expressed fear that he will die.
6. Will need to take consolidation and maintenance chemotherapy if a remission is achieved. This will require return to the cancer center on a regular schedule.
7. Sam will be hospitalized for at least another week to stabilize his condition and evaluate his status. He will then be discharged for recuperation at home.

Problem Approach	Strengths Approach
1., 4. Administer medications (e.g., Procrit). Check for signs of systemic infection or bleeding.	Same. If IM injections are needed, apply firm pressure for at least 5 minutes. Try to coordinate blood work so all is drawn at the same time. Blood or platelet transfusions may be needed. Discuss the need to avoid aspirin with Sam and Joyce.
2. Arrange for a nutritionist consult. Provide a high-calorie diet Provide medication after each diarrhea episode.	Diarrhea can lead to low blood potassium. Bananas have a high potassium content, and do not stimulate peristalsis. High fluid intake is desirable (also has an IV). Mouth sores require excellent mouth care and possible antibiotics. Monitor vital signs carefully. Work with a nutritionist to design a diet for the short-term and on discharge.
3. Encourage rest.	Reduce vital signs monitoring when asleep. Teach Sam how to do conditioning exercises while in bed to increase *capacity.*
5.–7. Reassure Sam that 70% of patients with AML achieve a complete remission after their first chemotherapy.	Foster a sense of hope by helping Sam to articulate *goals* for the short-term. Focus on *challenge* rather than threat. Enhance *capability* and *self-confidence* by teaching Sam and Joyce have to manage symptoms after discharge. Discuss choices that Sam can make to manage symptoms. Discuss Sam's preferences about enhancing *connections* with his children (and possibly arranging respite for Joyce). Inquire about Sam's desire for spiritual support. Sam needs to feel that he has some *control.* Reframing and instrumental support may be helpful.

Leddy Healthiness Scale

Leddy Healthiness Scale

Circle the number that best indicates your degree of agreement with each of the following statements. Please answer all of the questions the way you feel **right now**.

	Completely Agree	Mostly Agree	Slightly Agree	Slightly Disagree	Mostly Disagree	Completely Disagree
1. I think that I function pretty well.	6	5	4	3	2	1
2. I have goals that I look forward to accomplishing in the next year.	6	5	4	3	2	1
3. I am part of a close and supportive family.	6	5	4	3	2	1
4. I don't feel there is much that is meaningful in my life.	6	5	4	3	2	1
5. I have more than enough energy to do what I want to do.	6	5	4	3	2	1
6. I feel that I can accomplish anything I set out to do.	6	5	4	3	2	1
7. There is very little that I value in my life right now.	6	5	4	3	2	1
8. Having change(s) in my life makes me feel uncomfortable.	6	5	4	3	2	1
9. I have rewarding relationships with people.	6	5	4	3	2	1
10. I enjoy making plans for the future.	6	5	4	3	2	1
11. I feel free to choose actions that are right for me.	6	5	4	3	2	1
12. I feel like I've got little energy.	6	5	4	3	2	1
13. I am pleased to find that I am getting better with age.	6	5	4	3	2	1
14. I don't communicate much with family or friends.	6	5	4	3	2	1
15. I get excited thinking about new projects.	6	5	4	3	2	1
16. I feel good about my ability to influence change.	6	5	4	3	2	1
17. I'm not what you would call a goal oriented person.	6	5	4	3	2	1
18. I feel energetic.	6	5	4	3	2	1
19. I feel good about my freedom to make choices for my life.	6	5	4	3	2	1
20. I have a goal that I am trying to achieve.	6	5	4	3	2	1
21. I don't expect the future to hold much meaning for me.	6	5	4	3	2	1
22. I like exploring new possibilities.	6	5	4	3	2	1
23. I feel full of zest and vigor.	6	5	4	3	2	1
24. I feel fine.	6	5	4	3	2	1
25. I feel pretty sure of myself.	6	5	4	3	2	1
26. I feel isolated from people.	6	5	4	3	2	1

Page numbers followed by "f" denote figures; those followed by "t" denote tables

A

Accommodative coping, 51
Action stage, of change, 161–162, 165, 180t
Active coping, 116
Actual control, 90
Acupuncture, 136
Adaptation model, 120
Adaptation to threatening events, 35
Adherence to treatment, 177
Adipose tissue, 136
Adversity, 113
Affect, 4
Affective dimension, of hope, 39
Affiliative dimension, of hope, 39–40
Affirmative interactions, 65
African Americans
    culture of, 72–73
    identity among, 127
    personal control among, 99
    self-esteem needs, 127
    social support, 72–73, 127
Agency
    capability and, 83
    causal, 108–109
    commitment and, 48
    coping and, 99–100
    definition of, 37, 39, 83
    dependent-care, 80
    in Eastern cultures, 84
    environment and, 83
    influences on, 83
    perceived, 84
    requirements of, 83
    self agency, 79–80, 83
    self-care, 80–81, 84
    in Western cultures, 83–84, 86
Agent-ends relations, 90
Agent-means relations, 90
Anxious-ambivalence, 67
Approach goals, 48–49
Asian Americans
    culture of, 73–74
    helping relationships among, 175
    perceived control among, 100
    social support by, 73–74
Assessment
    cross-cultural, 10
    four front approach, 12–13
    health behavior change, 175
    psychological, 12
    strengths, 12–13

Assimilative coping, 51, 96
Attachment theory, 66–67
Attributional probing, 196
Autonomy, 96, 142
Autonomy support, 64
Avoidance, 67
Avoidance goals, 49–50
Avoidance style, of attachment, 66
Avoidant coping, 116
Awareness, 24

B

Bandura, Albert, 81–82
Beck's cognitive therapy, 53, 55
Behavior(s)
    health beliefs' effect on, 168
    influences on, 169
    self-efficacy and, 167
Behavior change. See Change; Health behavior
    change
Behavior goal model, 159, 169–170
Behavior modification, 176
Behavioral dimension, of hope, 39
Behavioral initiation, 163, 185
Behavioral maintenance, 185
Behavioral self-regulation, 98
Belief(s)
    changing of, 146–147
    competence, 90
    contingency, 90
    definition of, 168
    health, 168–169
    hope and, 40
Belonging, 65, 121
Belongingness hypothesis, 67
Benefit-finding, 35
Benefit-reminding, 35
Bonham-Cheney self-concept model,
    123–124
Brief negotiation model, 184–185
Broaden-and-build theory, 5–6

C

Capability
    agency and, 83
    definition of, 79
    requirements for, 80
    self-efficacy vs., 80
Capability theories
    Orem's self-care agency theory, 80–81
    self-determination theory, 81

Capacity
   components of, 132
   factors that decrease, 132
   interventions for, 136
Careative factors, 66
Catastrophizing, 54t
Causal agency, 108–109
Cell–cell communication, 135–136
Chakras, 133
Challenge
   adversity and, 113
   coping and, 113
   disposition toward, 112
   negative emotional reactions and, 113
   opportunities for success and, association
      between, 112–113
   overview of, 111–112
   physiological activity and, 113
   stress viewed as, 112
   theory of, 113–114
   threat and, 112
Challenge appraisals, 112
Chance expectations, 167
Change. *See also* Health behavior change
   barriers to, 166
   behavioral initiation/maintenance stage
      theory of, 163
   client-centered approach to, 162–163
   decisional balance regarding, 165–166
   energy and, 21
   motivation and, 49, 99
   personal control and, 193
   processes of, 162–165, 164t
   resistance to, 179
   self-schemas and, 123
   stages of, 160–162, 180t, 185–186
   transtheoretical model of, 156, 160–162,
      166–167, 179–182
   unpredictability of, 25
   views of, 2
Change talk, 184
Chaos theory, 6
Choice(s)
   decision-making vs., 105
   description of, 105
   interventions for generating, 109
   model of, 107
   quality of life and, 106
   values and, 106–107
Church-based health promotion, 175
Client-centered approach to change, 162–163
Client-nurse relationship, 20, 177–179,
   190–192
Cognitive dimension, of hope, 39

Cognitive distortions, 53t–55t
Cognitive restructuring, 181, 194
Cognitive theory, 156
Cognitive therapy, 53, 55
Cognitive-behavioral therapy, 41–42
Collarbone breathing procedure, 136
Collective control, 92
Collective self-esteem, 126
Collectivist culture, 144
Commitment, 48
Common sense model, 159
Communal mastery, 100
Communication, 192–193
Compensatory self-enhancement, 97
Competence
   control and, 93
   description of, 85
   multicultural, 85–86
Competence beliefs, 90
Complex tasks, 112
Complexity theory, 6
Component complexity, 112
Comprehensibility, 36
Conceptual competence, 85
Confidence. *See also* Self-esteem
   definition of, 120
   interventions for, 127–128
   model of, 120
   performance anxiety and, 120
   theory of, 120–121
Connectedness. *See also* Relatedness
   benefits of, 64
   interventions for creating, 76, 193
   overview of, 63–64
   religion and, 69–70
   social support and, 70–72
   spirituality and, 69–70
Connections
   description of, 26
   relatedness and, 64
Connections theories
   attachment theory, 66–67
   belongingness hypothesis, 67
   human relatedness theory, 68–69
   intimacy theory, 67–68
   physiological mechanisms, 68
   Watson's human science and human care
      theory, 66
Consciousness, 8
Consciousness raising, 164, 181, 194
Contemplation stage, of change, 161, 165, 180t,
   181
Contextual dimension, of hope, 40
Contingency, 93

Contingency beliefs, 90
Contingency contract, 177
Control
  actual, 90
  in African Americans, 99
  change and, 193
  collective, 92
  competence and, 93
  components of, 90
  contingency and, 93
  correlates of, 93–94
  demands and, 93
  descriptors for, 92–93
  global, 91
  in Healthiness Theory, 90
  illusion of, 91
  illusory, 92
  interpretive, 93
  interventions for, 100–101
  levels of, 93–94
  locus of. *See* Locus of control
  multicultural considerations, 99–100
  objective, 90, 92
  perceived, 90–92, 94
  personal, 90, 100–101
  predictive, 92–93
  primary, 92
  secondary, 92
  self-control, 92
  shared, 99
  situational, 90–91
  subjective, 92
  vicarious, 92–93
Control expectancy, 90
Control theories
  locus of control, 95–96
  Neuman's Health-Care Systems Model, 95
Controllability, 94
Coordinating complexity, 112
Coping
  accommodative, 51
  active, 116
  agency and, 99–100
  assimilative, 51, 96
  avoidant, 116
  challenge and, 113
  definition of, 96, 115
  effectiveness of, 42, 196
  emotion-focused, 97, 116
  function of, 96
  goals and, 51
  instrumental, 96
  positive outcomes of, 98

  preventive, 96
  proactive, 96–97, 115–116
  problem-focused, 96–97
  reactive, 96
  secondary, 92
  strategies for, 35, 56, 97
  stress and, 96–98, 116
  with threat, 112
  types of, 96–97
Counseling
  meaning-centered, 42–43
  patient-centered, 185
Counterconditioning, 164, 181–182
Countering, 195
Creativity, 107–108
Cross-cultural assessment, 10
Cultural appropriateness, 11–12
Cultural competency, 174–175
Cultural differences, 11
Cultural frame, 126
Cultural norms, 126–127
Cultural pluralism, 10
Cultural psychology, 143
Cultural relativism, 144
Cultural syndrome, 144–145
Culture. *See also* Eastern cultures; Multicultural competency; Western cultures
  of African Americans, 72–73
  of Asian Americans, 73–74
  collectivist, 144
  of Hispanic Americans, 73
  identity influenced by, 126
  Japanese, 74–75
  quality of life and, 151–152
  well-being influenced by, 143, 145
Cytokines, 136

D

Decisional balance, 165–166
Decision-making
  choice vs., 105
  factors that affect, 106
  family, 100
Deflection, 43–44
Demands, 93
Dependent-care agency, 80
Dialectical theory, 7–8
Dichotomous thinking, 53t
Disconnectedness, 68
Disengagement, 50
Dispositional optimism, 37, 56
Disqualifying the positive, 54t
Dopamine, 6
Dramatic relief, 164

Dynamic complexity, 112
Dynamical systems theory, 6

E

Eastern cultures. *See also* Culture; Multicultural
    competency
    agency in, 84
    competence in, 85–86
    description of, 10
    identity in, 126
    self in, 100
Efficacy expectations, 82, 166–167
Emotion(s)
    for coping with stress, 97
    cultural influences on, 9–10
    definition of, 4
    experiences associated with, 4
    hope and, 38–39
    multicultural competency and, 9–10
    negative, 5
    physiological theories of, 6–7
    positive
        description of, 5
        happiness and, 140–141
        perceived control and, 91
        stress-related physiological changes
            and, 6–7
    values and, 48
Emotional reasoning, 54t
Emotional support, 70
Emotion-focused coping, 97, 116
Enabling traits, 84
Enacted social support, 70
Ends, 26
Energetic healing, 135
Energetic patterning, 133
Energetic Patterning Nursing Practice Theory,
    133–135
Energy
    definition of, 21
    free, 21
    healthiness and, 28
    in Human Energy Model, 20–22
    mechanism of, 21
    metabolic, 132
    in physical body, 132–133
    of universal essence, 22f, 132
Energy field, 21, 132
Energy field vibration, 135
Energy healing, 134
Enmeshment, 68
Environment
    agency and, 83
    functional measures of, 151
    quality of life affected by, 149

structural measures of, 150–151
    of universal essence, 25
Environmental mastery, 141–142
Environmental reevaluation, 164, 181, 193
Environmental self-regulation, 98
Environmental stimuli, 120
Ethnocentric monoculturalism, 174
Events, 94
Existential meaning, 32–33
Existential psychology, 36
Expectancies, 55
Expectancy-value theories, 48, 55
Explanatory style
    bad events explained based on, 94
    hope, 37
    optimistic, 56
    pessimistic, 56
Extrinsic motivation, 49, 81
Eye roll treatment, 136

F

Family decision-making, 100
Fast-forwarding, 196
Feedback, 176
Field(s)
    attraction of, 21–22
    energy, 21, 132
    metabolic energy, 135–136
    universal essence, 21–22, 22f, 132–133
Flexibility, 25, 109
Floundering, 141
Flourishing, 141
Flow, 50–51, 114–115
Fortune telling, 54t
Four front approach, 12–13
Frankl, Viktor, 35, 43
Free energy, 21
Freedom, 105–106
Freedom of choice, 83
Free-flowing thinking, 8
Function-specific mastery, 93

G

Generalized hope, 38
Generativity, 33
Generic feedback, 176
Global control, 91
Global self-esteem, 126
Global-enhancement goals, 48
Glucose, 135
Goal(s)
    accomplishment of, 99
    achievement of, 51, 75, 197–198
    approach, 48–49
    avoidance, 49–50

coping and, 51
definition of, 48
global-enhancement, 48
group-enhancement, 48
interventions for, 75
intrinsic, 49
meaningful, 48
multicultural competency of, 57–58
mutual setting of, 51
nonconcordant, 52
optimism and, 55–56
overview of, 47–51
purpose and, 48
regulation of, 99
self-efficacy and, 51
self-enhancement, 48
strategies for attaining of, 59
unattainable, 49–50
values and, 48
well-being and, 143
Goal attainment theory, 51–52
Goal disengagement, 50
Goal engagement, 50
Goal orientation, 99
Goal re-engagement, 50
Goal theories
    Beck's cognitive therapy, 53, 55
    King's goal attainment theory, 51–52
    self-concordance model, 52, 52f
    self-determination theory, 53
Grand theory, 5
Group-enhancement goals, 48
Guided positive reappraisal, 14

H

Happiness
    satisfaction and, 140
    well-being and, 140
Hardiness, 142
Harmony/dissonance pattern, 25
Healing, 135
Health
    concept of, 25
    definition of, 25
    dominant model of, 2
    as expanding consciousness, 113–114
    interactions and, 68
    optimism and, correlation between, 57
    perception of, 140
    positive attributes of, 3
    positive responses for, 2
    relationships and, 65, 68
    social support and, 68, 70
    threats to, 2
    view of, 2

Health behavior change. *See also* Change
    advantages and disadvantages of, 165–166
    assessment in, 175
    barriers to, 166
    individual, 156
    initiation of, 187
    Internet programs for, 186–187
    model of, 159
    negative health trends and, 156
    resistance to, 179
    theories of
        characteristics of, 157t–158t
        criticism of, 160
        description of, 156
Health behavior change interventions
    adherence to treatment, 177
    behavior modification, 176
    description of, 176
    feedback, 176
    models of
        brief negotiation model, 184–185
        motivational interviewing, 182–184
        patient-centered counseling model, 185
        systems model of clinical preventive care, 179
        transtheoretical model, 179–182
    modifying and reinforcing treatment experience
        elements, 177
    nurse-client relationship, 177–179
    providing information, 177
    suggestions for, 187
Health behavior goal model, 159, 169–170
Health behaviors
    health beliefs' effect on, 168
    influences on, 169
    self-efficacy and, 167
Health belief model, 157t–158t, 166
Health beliefs, 168–169
Health disciplines, 3f
Health promotion
    church-based, 175
    description of, 3
Health promotion model, 169
Health realization theory, 8
Health-Care Systems Model, 95
Healthiness, 25–26
Healthiness Theory
    control in, 90
    description of, 5, 9, 20, 25–26
    empirical research based on, 27–28
    healthiness, 25–26
    links, 27t
    purpose in, 26
    tenets of, 26
Health-related quality of life, 150
Helicy, 107

Helping relationships, 164, 175, 181
Hierarchy of needs, 37
Hindus, 100
Hispanic Americans
    culture of, 73
    social support by, 73
Hope
    activities associated with, 38
    agency and, 37, 39
    approaches to, 37–38
    assessment of, 40–41
    beliefs and, 40
    characteristics of, 38
    components of, 40
    definition of, 38
    development of, 41
    dimensions of, 39
    dispositional optimism and, 37
    emotions and, 38–39
    explanatory style, 37
    generalized, 38
    objects of, 38
    particularized, 38
    spirituality and, 69
    Snyder's theory of, 39, 39f
    universal components of, 40
    well-being vs., 38–39
Hope therapy, 14
Human Becoming Theory, 34
Human being
    in Human Energy Model, 24
    structure of, 24
    unitary, 24
Human Energy Model
    awareness, 24
    concepts of, 22–25
    content of, 20
    description of, 20
    energy in, 20–22
    human being in, 24
    influences on, 20
    patterns, 24
    self-organization, 24
    structure of, 23f
Human essence, 134
Human science and human care theory, 66
Human strengths. See Strengths
Humor, 116
Hypothalamic-pituitary-adrenal axis, 7

I

Identity
    in African Americans, 127
    cultural influences on, 126
    in Eastern cultures, 126
    in Western cultures, 10, 126
Illusory control, 92
Imagery, 22
IMH, 5
Implicit self-esteem, 126
Indirect primary control, 92
Individualism, 57, 75, 145
Information, 21, 132
Information sharing, 194
Informational support, 70
Insecure attachment, 67
Insecurity, 67
Insight, 108
Instrumental coping, 96
Insulin, 135
Integrality, 107
Intentionality, 5
Interactions
    affirmative, 65
    definition of, 64
    health and, 68
    intimacy theory's view of, 68
Interdependence, 85
Internalization, 49
Internet programs, for health behavior change,
    186–187
Interpersonal attributes, 3
Interpersonal feedback, 176
Interpretive control, 93
Interventions
    description of, 14
    health behavior change. See Health behavior
        change interventions
    social support, 75–76, 193
    stress reduction, 196–198
    types of, 14–15
Intimacy theory, 67–68
Intrinsic motivation, 49, 81, 93

J

Japanese culture, 74–75

K

King's goal attainment theory, 51–52
Kovac's quality of life model, 149–150

L

Labeling, 55t
Languishing, 141
Learned optimism, 14
Leddy Healthiness Scale, 26–28
Life experiences model, 35–36

Life meaning, 33
Living matrix, 133
Locus of control
    description of, 95–96, 106
    internal, 167
    self-efficacy vs., 167–168
Logotherapy, 35, 43–44

M

Magical thinking, 42, 196
Maintenance stage, of change, 162–163, 165, 180t
Manageability, 36, 98
Marcus and Kitayama well-being model, 143
Maslow's hierarchy of needs, 37
Mastery
    communal, 100
    description of, 82
    environmental, 141–142
    function-specific, 93
    role-specific, 93
Matter, 21, 132
Maximization, 54t
May's theory, 37
Meaning
    characteristics of, 32
    creation of, 32
    definition of, 32
    description of, 24
    existential, 32–33
    interventions for developing
        cognitive-behavioral therapy, 41–42
        five-step approach, 43
        logotherapy existential psychotherapy,
            43–44
        meaning-centered counseling, 42–43
    life, 33
    purpose and, 32
    relational, 97
    search for, 52
    situational, 32
    sources of, 33
Meaning models and theories
    adaptation to threatening events, 35
    existential psychology, 36
    Human Becoming Theory, 34
    life experiences model, 35–36
    logotherapy, 35
    Maslow's hierarchy of needs, 37
    May's theory, 37
    sense of coherence, 36–37
Meaning-as-comprehensibility, 32
Meaning-as-significance, 32
Meaning-centered counseling, 42–43
Meaningful goals, 48

Meaningful life, 33
Meaningful purpose, 50
Meaningfulness, 26, 33, 36–37
Means-ends relations, 90
Metabolic energy, 132
Metabolic energy field, 135–136
Mind, 8
Mind reading, 54t
Minimization, 54t
Model theory, 5
Modified health belief model, 159
Moods, 4
Motivation
    change and, 49, 99
    description of, 193–194
    expectancy-value models of, 48
    extrinsic, 49, 81
    intrinsic, 49, 81, 93
    needs and, alignment between, 37
    opponent theory of, 7
    values' effect on, 107
Motivational interviewing, 182–184
Multicultural competence, 85–86
Multicultural competency. See also Culture
    control, 99–100
    cross-cultural assessment, 10
    description of, 9
    emotions and, 9–10
    ethnocentric monoculturalism, 174
    goals, 57–58
    requirements for, 10
    self, 99–100
    social support, 72–75
    well-being, 144–145
Mutuality, 69

N

Nadis, 133
Native Americans, 74
"Need to belong," 191
Needs
    hierarchy of, 37
    motivation and, alignment between, 37
Negative affect, 4
Negative emotions, 5
Negative mood, 4
Nervous system, 135–136
Neuman's Health-Care Systems Model, 95
Neuropeptides, 7
Newman's theory of health as expanding
    consciousness, 113–114
Nine-gamut treatments, 136
Nonconcordant goals, 52
Noninvasive therapies, 134t

North American Nursing Diagnosis Association, 134
Nurse-client communication, 192–193
Nurse-client relationship, 20, 177–179, 190–192
Nursing
    basis for, 25
    goal of, 120
    purpose of, 20
Nursing practice, strengths-based, 190

O

Obesity, 156
Objective control, 90, 92
Operational traits, 84
Opponent theory of motivation, 7
Optimism
    definition of, 55
    dispositional, 37, 56
    explanatory style, 56
    goals and, 55–56
    health and, correlation between, 57
    interventions for, 58–59
    longevity and, 141
    pessimism vs., 56–57
Optimism training, 58–59
Orem's self-care agency theory, 80–81
Oscillation, 21
Outcome expectancies, 166
Outcome expectation, 82
Overgeneralization, 53t
Oxytocin, 6

P

Paradoxical intention, 43
Parallelism, 68
Parse's Human Becoming Theory, 34
Particularized hope, 38
Pathways thinking, 39
Patient-centered counseling model, 185
Patterns
    definition of, 24
    harmony/dissonance, 25
Perceived agency, 84
Perceived barriers, 168
Perceived benefits, 168
Perceived consequences, 168
Perceived control
    among Asian Americans, 100
    description of, 90–92
    religion and, 100
    work experiences and, 94
Perceived relational value, 121
Perceived self-efficacy, 82, 84, 166, 168
Perceived severity, 168

Perceived social support, 70
Perceived state, 99
Perceived susceptibility, 168
Perceived threat, 168
Performance anxiety, 120
Performance competence, 85
Personal control, 90, 100–101
Personal growth, 50, 142–143
Personal identity
    cultural influences on, 126
    description of, 123–124
Personal self-regulation, 98
Personal traits, 84
Personalization, 55t
Personalized feedback, 176
Perturbations, 136
Pessimism
    interventions for, 58
    multicultural considerations, 57–58
    optimism vs., 56–57
Pessimistic explanatory style, 56
Physical body, 132
Physical closeness, 74
Positive affect, 4
Positive beliefs, 3
Positive comparisons, 99
Positive emotions
    description of, 5
    happiness and, 140–141
    perceived control and, 91
    stress-related physiological changes and, 6–7
Positive functioning, 3
Positive reappraisal, 14, 194
Possible selves, 122–123
Power, in Theory of Healthiness, 26
Precontemplation stage, of change, 161, 163, 165, 180t
Predictability, 94
Predictive control, 92–93
Preoccupation style, of attachment, 67
Preparation stage, of change, 161, 165, 180t
Presence, 34
Preventive care, 179
Preventive coping, 96
Primary control, 92
Proactive coping, 96–97, 115–116
Problem-focused coping, 96–97
Procedural competence, 85
Process theory, 144
Processing-thinking, 8
Protection motivation theory, 157t–158t
Psychological assessment, 12
Psychological functioning, 142
Psychological well-being, 108, 142–143
Psychotherapy, logotherapy existential, 43–44

Purpose
    development of, 35
    goals and, 48
    in Healthiness Theory, 26
    meaning and, 32
    meaningful, 50
    in Ryff's psychological well-being model, 142
    sense of, 35
Purposive supplication, 92

Q

Quality of life
    components of, 147
    cultural considerations, 151–152
    environmental factors of, 149
    health-related, 150
    interventions for, 151–152
    Kovac's model of, 149–150
    models of, 147–148
    social production functions theory of, 150
    social support and, 150–151
    societal/environmental perspective of, 148–149

R

Racism, 174
Rapport building, 183, 191
Rapprochement, 167
Reactance theory, 184
Reactive coping, 96
Recall, 177, 194
Reciprocity, 69
Reframing, 194–195
Reinforcement management, 164, 182
Relapse stage, of change
    description of, 165, 180t
    prevention of, 185–186
Relatedness. *See also* Connectedness
    activities that contribute to, 191
    autonomy support and, 64
    connection and, 64
    definition of, 68
    description of, 49
    interventions for, 74–75
    in Japanese culture, 74
    levels of, 64–65
    social processes associated with, 68–69
    states of, 65
    theory of, 68–69
Relational attributes, 3
Relational meaning, 97
Relationship(s)
    definition of, 65
    healing, 164
    health and, 65, 68
        helping, 175, 181
        life satisfaction and, 65
        nurse-client, 20, 177–179, 190–192
        supportive, 71
Relaxation therapies, 14, 196
Religion
    benefits of, 69–70
    description of, 37
    perceived control affected by, 100
    spirituality vs., 69
Religious faith, 11
Resilience, 114
Resonance, 21
Resonancy, 107
Revised health promotion model, 159, 169
Rogers' Science of Unitary Human Beings, 107
Role-specific mastery, 93
ROPES model, 13
Rotter's social learning theory, 157t–158t
Roy's adaptation model, 120
Ryff's psychological well-being model, 142–143

S

Satisfaction, 140
Schema assessment, 124–125
Schema model, of self-concept, 123
Schemata, 144
Science of Unitary Human Beings, 107
Secondary control, 92
Secure style, of attachment, 67
Selective abstraction, 53t
Selective attribution, 99
Selective ignoring, 99
Selective valuation, 99
Self, 100
Self conceptions, 122
Self-acceptance, 142
Self-actualization, 64
Self-agency
    description of, 79–80, 83
    environments that affect, 83
Self-awareness, 196
Self-care agency, 80–81, 84
Self-concept
    Bonham-Cheney model of, 123–124
    definition of, 121
    description of, 97
    positive, 121–122
    possible selves, 122–123
    schema model of, 123
    status dynamic approach to, 124
    working, 122
Self-concordance model, 52, 52f
Self-confidence. *See* Confidence

Self-control, 92, 136
Self-definition, 36
Self-determination model of well-being, 108–109
Self-determination theory, 53, 81
Self-efficacy
    capability vs., 80
    characteristics of, 81–82
    competence and, 85
    definition of, 80–82
    goals and, 51
    health behaviors associated with, 167
    information sources that affect, 82–83
    locus of control and, 96
    locus of control vs., 167–168
    manipulations of, 167
    outcomes of, 83
    perceived, 82, 84, 166, 168
    self-regulation and, 82
Self-efficacy theory, 159, 166–167
Self-enhancement goals, 48
Self-esteem. *See also* Confidence
    in African Americans, 127
    antecedents to, 125
    collective, 126
    definition of, 125
    description of, 70
    distortions in, 127
    in females vs. males, 125, 127
    global, 126
    implicit, 126
    interventions for, 127–128
    labels associated with, 125–126
    sense of belonging and, 121
    state, 126
    trait, 125–126
    well-being and, 145
Self-fulfilling prophecies, 91
Self-healing, 135
Self-liberation, 164, 181
Self-organization, 24
Self-perspective, 124
Self-reevaluation, 164, 181, 193
Self-regulation, 82, 98–99, 122, 136
Self-schemas, 123
Self-talk, 128
Sense of belonging, 65, 121
Sense of coherence, 36–37, 94, 98
Sense-making, 35
Shared control, 99
"Should" statements, 54t
Signature strengths, 9
Situational control, 90–91
Situational meaning, 32
Situation-specific social support, 70

Social cognitive theory, 81–82
Social learning theory
    Bandura's, 95, 157t–158t
    Rotter's, 157t–158t
Social liberation, 164, 181
Social persuasion, 82–83
Social production functions, 150
Social support
    by African Americans, 72–73, 127
    by Asian Americans, 73–74
    assessment of, 71–72
    components of, 71
    connectedness and, 70–72
    definition of, 70
    emotional, 70
    enacted, 70
    health and, 68, 70
    by Hispanic Americans, 73
    informational, 70
    interventions for, 75–76, 193
    in Japanese culture, 74–75
    multicultural considerations, 72–75
    by Native Americans, 74
    perceived, 70
    promotion of, 196
    quality of life and, 150–151
    from relationships, 71
    situation-specific, 70
    stress reaction and, 71, 151
Society
    quality of life based on, 148–149
    values based on, 144
Sociometer Theory, 120–121
Spirituality, 11
Sporadic writing, 49
State self-esteem, 126
Status dynamic view, of self-concept, 124
Stimulus control, 164, 181
Strengths
    assessment of, 12–13
    classification systems for, 8–9
    definition of, 8
    descriptions of, 2, 4
    health promotion focus on, 3
    nursing practice based on, 190
    promotion of, 14–15
    questions and issues regarding, 15
    ROPES model for assessing, 13
    signature, 9
    terms used to describe, 4
Strengths perspective, 4
Strengths theories
    broaden-and-build theory, 5–6
    dialectical theory, 7–8
    dynamical systems theory, 6

health realization theory, 8
IMH, 5
opponent theory of motivation, 7
overview of, 5
physiological theories, 6–7
Stress
as challenge, 112
cognitive appraisal processes and, 112
coping and, 96–98, 116
definition of, 111–112
positive outcomes of confronting, 98
reduction of, 196–198
relational nature of, 111
social support and, 71, 151
Stressor, 151
Structuralist-behaviorist approach, to
spirituality, 69
Structure, 24
Subjective control, 92
Subjective well-being, 140–141
Support. *See* Social support
Support schemas, 71
Supportive communication, 193
Supportive relationships, 71
Supportive transactions, 71
Synchronization, 21
Synchronized dynamic interaction, 21
Synchrony, 69
Snyder's hope theory, 39, 39f
Systems model of clinical preventive care,
179

T

Tailored feedback, 176
Targeted feedback, 176
Teaching, 194
Temporal dimension, of hope, 40
Termination stage, of change, 162, 165
Theories. *See also specific theory*
capability, 80–81
challenge, 113–114
confidence, 120 121
connections. *See* Connections theories
control, 95–96
definition of, 5
goal. *See* Goal theories
grand, 5
meaning. *See* Meaning models and theories
model, 5
self-efficacy, 159, 166–167
Theory of health locus of control, 159
Theory of Healthiness. *See* Healthiness Theory
Theory of locus of control, 159
Theory of Participation, 20

Theory of planned behaviour
characteristics of, 157t–158t
description of, 159
Theory of reasoned action
characteristics of, 157t–158t
description of, 159
health beliefs in, 168
Therapeutic interviewing, 191
Therapeutic relationship, 14
Therapeutic touch, 22
Thinking
agency, 39
dichotomous, 53t
free-flowing, 8
magical, 42, 196
pathways, 39
processing-thinking, 8
reframing of, 195
Thought(s)
changing of, 146–147
description of, 8
Thought field therapy, 136
Threats
coping with, 112
perceived, 168
resilience as adaptive response to, 114
Time frame alteration, 99
Trait, 4
Trait self-esteem, 125–126
Transcendent approach, to spirituality, 69
Transtheoretical model, 156, 160–162, 166–167,
179–182
Treatment adherence, 177
Turning point, 7

U

Unattainable goals, 49–50
Undoing hypothesis, 6
Unitary human beings, 24
Universal essence
description of, 20–22, 22f, 132
environment of, 25
Universal essence field, 132–133

V

Validation, 64
Value guidance approach, to spirituality, 69
Values
choice and, 106–107
definition of, 106
emotions and, 48
motivational effects of, 107
societal differences, 144
Vicarious control, 92–93

Virtues, 8–9
Vital energy
    definition of, 132
    nursing practice theory based on, 133–135
    structure of, 132–133
Vitality, 132

W

"Wake-up call," 97–98
Watson's human science and human care
    theory, 66
Waves, 21, 132
Well-being
    changing thoughts and beliefs to increase,
        146–147
    components of, 140
    cultural differences in, 143, 145
    economic influences, 145
    happiness and, 140
    hope vs., 38–39
    interventions for, 145–147
    Marcus and Kitayama model of, 143

multicultural considerations, 144–145
national differences in, 145
Oishi's goal approach to, 143
patterns of, 141
process theory of, 144
psychological, 108, 142–143
quality of life and. See Quality of life
relationships and, 65
Ryff's psychological well-being model,
    142–143
self-determination model of, 108–109
self-esteem and, 145
subjective, 140–141
Well-being therapy, 145–146
Western cultures. See also Culture; Multicultural
    competency
    agency in, 83–84, 86
    competence in, 85
    description of, 10, 83–84
    identity in, 10, 126
    self in, 100
Willpower, 136
Working self-concept, 122

About the Author

Susan Kun Leddy earned a bachelor of science in nursing from Skidmore College, Saratoga, New York, in 1960, a master of science in nursing (teaching medical-surgical nursing) from Boston University in 1965, a doctor of philosophy (nursing science) from New York University in 1973, and did post-doctoral work at Harvard University (1985) and the University of Pennsylvania (1986-98).

Dr. Leddy initially taught in diploma schools of nursing for 4 years and then in the baccalaureate program at Columbia University before completing doctoral work. She was then one of four founding faculty for the RN-BSN program at Pace University. In 1976, after a year as an NLN consultant, she was asked to do a feasibility study and then write the proposal to the State of New York for a new RN-BSN program at Mercy College. She became the first chairperson of the program, which opened in 1977.

Dr. Leddy left Mercy College in 1981 to first become dean of the School of Nursing, and then dean of the reconstituted College of Health Sciences at the University of Wyoming. In 1988, she became dean of the School of Nursing at Widener University, returning to teaching primarily in the doctoral program there in 1993. She is now a professor emerita in the School of Nursing.

In addition to authoring *Health Promotion: Mobilizing Human Strengths to Enhance Health, Wellness, and Well-Being,* Dr. Leddy is the co-author with Lucy Hood of *Conceptual Bases of Professional Nursing,* 6th edition (2006), *Integrative Health Promotion: Conceptual Bases for Nursing Practice,* 2nd edition (2006), and is working on a manuscript, Nursing Knowledge and Nursing Science, with Jacqueline Fawcett. She has authored numerous periodical publications, and is actively engaged in research.

Dr. Leddy has two daughters, Deborah, who is finishing the veterinary medicine program at the University of Pennsylvania, and Erin, who is a student in the Master's degree in Social Work Program at West Chester University in Pennsylvania. Her granddaughter, Katie, was born October 12, 2001.

Dr. Leddy is an avid traveler, especially to exotic places (most recently Bhutan, West Africa, China, and Cambodia). She also knits, weaves, does creative writing, is re-learning bridge, and dabbles in watercolor painting.

3